Fourteen Doors And A Mattress

GAIL WENCH

AuthorHouse™
1663 Liberty Drive
Bloomington, IN 47403
www.authorhouse.com
Phone: 1-800-839-8640

This book is a work of non-fiction. Unless otherwise noted, the author and the publisher
make no explicit guarantees as to the accuracy of the information contained in this book
and in some cases, names of people and places have been altered to protect their privacy.

© 2010 Gail Wench. All rights reserved.

No part of this book may be reproduced, stored in a retrieval system, or
transmitted by any means without the written permission of the author.

First published by AuthorHouse 3/2/2010

ISBN: 978-1-4490-8687-9 (e)
ISBN: 978-1-4490-8686-2 (sc)

Library of Congress Control Number: 2010901879

Printed in the United States of America
Bloomington, Indiana

This book is printed on acid-free paper.

Book Cover illustrated by Jacqueline McKeown
Photo of author by Lonna Sullivan

For My John who has been with me through it all.

FOREWARD

"You must do the thing you think you cannot do".

- Eleanor Roosevelt

I always said, "I am not afraid to die. But I don't want to be sick and suffer." Instead, I hoped I would be run over by a truck and die instantly. My terrible fear of hospitals and even visiting family and friends made me nauseous.

Don't let me scare you off; this is not a book just about illness. It has more to do with desperation, determination, hope, and courage during the most terrifying year and a half of my life.

As an American History teacher, I would preface each new school year by saying to my students, "What we are going to read, study, and discuss is all true to the best of our knowledge." For example, I explained, "If we take an incident that was witnessed by five people, each person will have a slightly different interpretation of what they believe to be "the truth". In fact, in time the story may actually become distorted. Textbooks, newspapers, and biographies most likely are never 100% accurate. So it is that we sometimes learn to take our newly learned information with a grain of salt, like you, dear readers, as you travel along the path of my journey.

To the best of my knowledge, my account and interpretation are true. Admittedly prejudice in some ways, yet I don't apologize, for what I have written is how I viewed the circumstances.

Contents

Foreward   vii

1. Fate or Foolishness   1
2. Everything is Relative   5
3. The Onset   11
4. Hope, Wine and The MRI   15
5. Mumbo Jumbo   21
6. What are the Odds?   27
7. Just Do It   33
8. The Vulture   39
9. At Last   43
10. Grasping at Straws   49
11. The Thief of Time   55
12. Mountain Climbing   59
13. Fourteen Doors and a Mattress   65
14. Movin' On   69
15. Head Case   73
16. My Twelve Days of Christmas   75
17. Doctor Gorgeous   79
18. The Mask   83
19. On the Brighter Side   87

20. Enough is Enough   91

21. Mixed Emotions   93

22. Turning Point   99

23. Celebration   101

24. Hallehujah   103

25. Blink   105

26. Not for Sissies   107

27. Déjà Vu   109

28. What's Up Doc?   113

29. It's Not Over   115

30. Od'ed On Yoga   119

31. Living in the Now   123

32. Finding Balance   127

33. Is Life Beautiful?   129

34. A Serendipitous Journey   131

Epilogue   135

Chapter 1
FATE OR FOOLISHNESS

As one of those people who believe everything happens for a reason, fate plays an important role in my life. I'm always wondering why a certain person or a particular event comes into my life. How will it affect me, should I go along with the idea, should I pursue the course; what if I don't? And most importantly, do I really have the freedom of choice or is this destined as well?

Recently watching the movie *Grand Canyon,* my feelings were supported by Kevin Kline's character, Mac, who receives help from the stranger, Danny Glover, as Simon, who rescues Mac from a soon to be nasty mugging. It was destiny Mac knows that brought the kind, unknown guy to his aid. Not seeing it that way at all, Simon chalks it up to just an inconsequential event.

When Mac tries to convince him by relating another incident when he was saved by a stranger while jay walking across the road called the "Miracle Mile", Simon laughs it off, but asks, "Hey, pal, ever been to the Grand Canyon?" "Never, but I've always been meaning to," Mac acknowledged. "You know Mac, we're mere specks and so small compared to the Grand Canyon. Don't take yourself so seriously."

In the last scene of the film, Mac and his wife, with their adopted baby (another fateful event in Mac's life), and Simon and his girlfriend, are standing at an overlook of the Grand Canyon. "Not all bad," Mac utters, as the camera sweeps the width and depth of this spectacular, awesome and powerful site, transcending the experiences of all that have the chance to view it. Overwhelmed by the beauty, size and timelessness of the Grand Canyon make us aware of our short, earthly existence, and, like Simon, of our miniscule and insignificant roles. Look at the big picture; don't sweat the small things.

Shall we go with the flow? Or, if you are looking for something, will you go to every length to find it? Will you answer the call? If you believe there is an answer to everything you will.

After finishing a delicious dinner at Gurney's Inn in April of 1993, my husband, John and I took a short stroll on their 'beautiful wide, white, sandy beach' before beginning our drive back home. Just before we left, we stopped at the Spa pavilion and overheard a woman mention she needed a ride to Amagansett to catch the Hampton Jitney to Manhattan. We also learned she was an astrologer who worked at Gurney's on the weekends. "Should we ask her if she'd like us to drop her off since we're going that way?" John asked me. "Sure, maybe we'll hear an interesting story!"

As soon as we all settled in our car, John asked the question I almost blurted out, "So, how did you become interested in astrology?" Shelley entertained us with a pretty predicable account of how she read a lot about astrology and before long, friends were asking her questions. Little by little, she became more involved to where astrology readings were added to her singing, dancing and comedic repertoire. Now having just landed a part in the soap opera, "A Guiding Light", she would have to prioritize. A delightful 35-40 year old woman, pleasingly plump with long golden hair and sparkling gold eye shadow, who wore a black knit outfit, seemed to fit life on the stage.

By the time we reached Amagansett, we got to know Shelley pretty well, but were surprised when she told us she had visited Montauk several times but had never been to Gurney's before she "got the call". "What call?" John asked quickly. "Well," began Shelley, "I was sitting on the beach one day last summer looking out at the ocean and the ocean whispered to me, 'go to Gurney's and do astrology.' In a flash, John said, "You mean you actually heard the ocean speak to you; please explain."

Shelley thought for a moment and said slowly, "Well, it wasn't actually a 'voice' as much as it was something in my heart that told me. We all have the power to hear things like this if we listen closely enough. Sitting there quietly, listening to the rustling sounds of the waves, something definitely spoke to me."

"It happened to Gail once," John said. "She heard something in her heart about a year ago."

Before John continued, we had arrived at the Jitney stop. We exchanged phone numbers and I told Shelley I would like to have a reading with her at Gurney's someday. "Be sure to know your exact birth time," she smiled and waved.

On the drive home, I kept thinking about Shelley and was comforted knowing I wasn't alone in having something in my heart. Somehow chatting with Shelley confirmed what I already knew.

Chapter 2
EVERYTHING IS RELATIVE

John and I have been married for nineteen years. We have no children. When most people describe us as a couple who look good together, I laugh, but I think so, too! The longer we are together, the more we will probably look alike but in reality we are quite opposite. Tall and with dark hair and a ready smile, John has a bit of mischief about him to which people are drawn and his friendly manner and chattiness add to his charm. As a Sales Supervisor, he is tops! No, John isn't a professional but he is a tremendous asset to his company. How fortunate I am to benefit from John's work ethics and his genuine kindness and ongoing supportive ways toward me.

At 5' 6" I can wear heels with John! Some gals I know are frustrated with short husbands. And since I am probably a little too concerned with how I look, the fact that I am blond, have a tall man, delights me. In the last few years, clothes and jewelry have become very important to me. Maybe the saying "Clothes Make the Man" is very true, for shopping and planning my outfits each day and hearing lots of compliments have definitely rewarded me!

An easy life style where John and I can both fulfill our days productively apart makes the times we are together even more special.

5

After graduating from college in the early 1970's, the job market for teachers on Long Island was dismal and I substituted for a year and a half before landing a kindergarten position in Lindenhurst, my home town. Even though teaching was wonderful, it was impossible to remain in the same grade or school for very long due to the declining enrollments, and after seven years of teaching on the elementary level I was "excessed" with no hopes for another position in the near future.

After a two year hiatus during which time I even thought of finding a new career, a high school friend encouraged me to look into jobs on the secondary level. At first I thought the idea was crazy since my experience was with much younger elementary students, and truthfully, I was also afraid, yet something (maybe desperation) made me pursue her advice. If I don't like it, I'll just quit I told myself!

It was amazing, that someone like me, afraid of her own shadow, proved to the school administrators, the students, and most of all to myself that I could handle it! Lesson learned; don't ever say never until you've tried. And so, way back in 1981, I reinvented myself as a Junior High Social Studies teacher, teaching five periods a day, supervised a homeroom and had a duty period. My colleagues understood when I would tell them we were actors with five stage shows a day! Our jobs were hectic but the hours were from 8am to 3pm and the vacations, especially the summer ones, were fantastic!

As time went on, I enjoyed the secondary level even more and kept advancing my grasp of American History. My rapport with the kids was special, just as there was something memorable going on in my classroom almost on a daily basis. And since 7th and 8th grades usually are the most difficult grades for the children, I felt extremely fortunate to make the impact I did.

Working along with the eighty different personalities of my colleagues gave me the opportunity to laugh or commiserate during my breaks. Indeed, the faculty became an important part of my life as did my students. Yet, there were times when I felt my job "swallowed me up and spit me out". As soon as I awoke each day, I began thinking of my lessons and before I fell asleep every night I'd be planning the next day's classroom adventure. Even though I knew I was "overdoing and overloading" so to speak, it was the only way I knew how; give it my all.

In 1988 rumblings of financial cutbacks and lay offs spread. Slowly but surely I became the "bottom man" on the seniority list.

What are the odds that with over 700 teachers in the district who have fifteen to sixteen years of experience I would be one of the twelve teachers let go? In February 1991, I was summoned to the superintendent's office and given my 30 day notice. There were no provisions for job security even with the union; the political bullshit "sacrificed twelve sacrificial lambs".

I cried, I screamed, I carried on like a martyr but in the end I left quietly. My broken heart could not allow me to face my students and say my last good-byes. The note John left for me the following morning after I cried all night long said, "I know things will work out. I heard it from a good Source. Love, John." I cried for another hour.

During my first empty, quiet weeks ahead I discovered that human nature fell into two main categories. Either one was a warm, caring, understanding, person or a selfish, thoughtless jerk. Some people (guardian angels, I called them) came out of nowhere to support me while others were rude and cruel. Guardian angels like Bea, my walking buddy colleague, who had been a walker for years, and who had become a dear friend over the years, called me from school every few days. We would often meet to walk for "old time's sake".

Soon, by chance, another "walking buddy" came into my life. An English teacher, one of the "lambs" with whom I was acquainted, agreed to meet me for a trek to the unemployment office and then take a walk. A wonderful gal who loved to walk and who didn't have a partner was delighted, and so, little by little our friendship and the miles we accrued turned out to be one of my most emotionally and physically satisfying adventures. I was amazed that Katie was not really upset about losing her position; in fact, she relished it and thought of it as an opportunity since she could spend a lot more time with her 4 year old son.

Why couldn't I change the way I looked at things, I wondered? If it hadn't been for Katie, I know I would have continued my self-designed painful existence. I began to realize that I was wasting time worrying when I could redirect my thoughts and make this time in my life pleasurable. Instead of focusing on what had happened, maybe I thought, just maybe, there was some sort of cosmic reasoning for all this.

"Do not worry" became my mantra and soon I actually looked forward to and planned normal happy activities. John and I accepted my parent's invitation to meet them in Puerto Rico for a week. What wonders that vacation did for my attitude!

In June 1991, four months after my lay off, I learned there was a retirement incentive being initiated and several Social Studies teachers were taking advantage of it, leaving several openings!

Oh my God, I would be going back in September! Not only returning but returning to my same building and same room (112c)! My principal, Joe Pisano and my Department Chairman, Jack, two great guys, helped me through this adjustment period.

Chapter 3

THE ONSET

"I got my life back!" It didn't take long to get back to my old routine. The kids were great, some very nice new teachers were on board, Bea and I walked during our daily break and all was right with the world! Everything was as it should be.

Then on January 10th, 1992, my life took a very different direction. It all began innocently enough when after a nice, relaxing two week Christmas vacation, I told Bea during our chilly winter walk, that I ate so much during the holidays but was so excited to return to school and that I hadn't slept well the previous night; the usual chit chat. After another exercise walk after school with Laurie, colleague and friend, I knew for sure I would sleep like a rock that night!

However, as soon as I came home I felt strange aches and pains and actual muscle twitches in my legs. "That's what you get from overdoing your walking," I scolded myself. When these odd spasms continued for about a week, I decided to make a doctor's appointment. Dr. Mary Mathias, a lovely young physician with a promising career, diagnosed my situation due to a pinched nerve in my back, and suggested more tests and physical therapy. "How about a chiropractor?" I asked. "Okay," she replied, "but watch who you go to."

11

Explaining that I knew one I had seen a few years ago when I hurt my back, and liked very much, she had no objections.

Looking forward to seeing "my chiropractor" again and recalling how patient and interested he was in helping me, I felt I was surely on the right track, and since my appointments were three times a week, I got to know Shari, his receptionist very well, too.

Just as if it was old home week, Dr. B and Shari greeted me warmly. Getting right down to business, Dr. B began with X-rays and an examination. Usually a pinched nerve, he explained, would cause a problem in one leg, not both, and on one area, not up and down both legs, and mentioned the possibility of a more serious cause such as multiple sclerosis; a possibility I brushed away. For the time being I was told not to do exercise walking during the three times a week he would be treating me. If I continued to have pain, he would refer me to a specialist.

Determined to rid myself of whatever it was I had, three of my lunch periods each week, were spent at physical therapy. Bea was a real good sport and understood my "forced holiday". We would resume our walking soon, of that I was sure.

By the end of January, my legs were "twitching" and the pain continued. It was as if my legs made me tired. Finally, deciding to walk now and then, I noticed that my legs were better, yet when at rest, the pain returned and the twitching was out of control!

John and I had made plans to vacation at Gurney's Inn (our favorite LI spot) during the mid-winter break. What better place to walk I felt! However, my first walk turned into another sleepless night. A day at the Spa rejuvenated me; the sauna, the massage, a sea salt body scrub and a manicure and pedicure was just "what the doctor ordered". Swimming in the indoor salt water pool, eating beside the huge windows, overlooking the ocean, was just what I called "heaven on earth". Little did I know or could have even thought in my wildest imagination that I would not return to this paradise until my path would take me on a long journey through hell.

In March, severe pains in both hip joints didn't seem to concern Dr. B at first; "a touch of bursitis," he maintained. When the pains increased, he decided to order blood work, a urine test, and an MRI of my lower back. Agreeing to the blood tests but shying away from the MRI, I was anxious to hear the blood results a few days later.

Dressed in a navy and white two piece suit with navy stockings and shoes, I rushed to his office during my lunch break and waited on pins and needles until he ushered me into his office. My white blood cell count was a little high and ketones were found in my urine, he informed me, and made it very clear that I was to go to my medical doctor right away. The look on my face, I'm sure he remembers to this day, for not only was I scared and worried but I actually felt I would be sick right then and there. Fortunately, Shari intervened and called Dr. Mathias, but the soonest available appointment was for the next day.

My anxiety and physical pain were such that I could not finish out the day at school and asked to leave early. As soon as I got home, I called my old family doctor, a little Taiwanese man, whom I hadn't seen in years (had no need to). He took me right away and put me at ease when he told me not to be concerned since he didn't feel the blood count was too high and the ketone situation was okay. After his examination, his diagnosis was of a pinched nerve in my back which caused the leg problems with possible arthritis in both hips. Insisting on an MRI, however, I reluctantly agreed. His prescription for an anti-inflammatory, I took but a few times, since I was "living on Anacin".

For the first time in my career, my mind was not on my teaching, for I was consumed by what seemed to be my deteriorating health. In fact, on a half day of school for the students and an afternoon session for the faculty, when we assembled in the cafeteria for a guest speaker, whose purpose was to educate the general public on becoming aware of those with severe physical difficulties, my ears stood at attention. She pointed out how just about anyone could become a victim. Sometimes certain afflictions will go away, she said, other times one is stuck with them for life. She emphasized the fact that one's entire life can change in an instant. My sick feeling reaction, I knew, was because she was talking directly to me! It was at this moment I knew that I was in for something serious. That day, dressed in my deep purple suit with a print satin blouse, and a much admired gold rope chain, stuck in my mind like something that gets caught in your throat. I will never forget it.

Chapter 4

HOPE, WINE AND THE MRI

No longer walking for exercise, I began to hang out in the faculty room during my breaks where there was always lots of friendly chatter, coffee and a comfortable place to unwind. Soon Hope, a young, energetic teacher and I became very friendly. At twenty four she was so enthusiastic, warm and had a wonderful sense of humor! We sure hit it off right away; another dose of much needed medicine for me. Hope would often drop by my classroom. We were like college students keeping up with the latest buzz. She was between boyfriends, which made our get-togethers easy and frequent.

There were times, however, that I just could not physically do all the things we planned to do. It was Hope who volunteered to take me to my first MRI appointment. Magnetic Resonance Imagery was a fairly newly developed piece of equipment that operated without the harmful effects of radiation to take the image of one's insides.

The description alone scared the life out of me, so before I made a definite appointment, I called the office and explained my claustrophobia. "But the sides will be open, dear, in front of you and behind you." One of my friends suggested I take Valium. "No way, pills and I don't mix," I almost shouted! Then out of the blue, one of my "guardian angel" school

15

chums, Marianne said, "If you want to relax, Gail, why don't you drink some wine just before the test?" Now, how brilliant was Marianne?

Needless to say I worried all week, but as John, Hope and I arrived at the parking lot on MRI Day, I broke open my coveted bottle of white wine and filled the paper cup almost to the brim. In roughly five minutes, I had swallowed 2 cups of wine, and my lips felt numb.

John and Hope thought I walked a pretty straight line from the car to the "den of terror." As soon as I appeared in a blue paper gown, John and Hope giggled and teased me before we all walked into THAT ROOM.

Immediately, the technician slid out a cot to put me on as I tore part of my gown, taped my feet together, and before I could utter a single word, the cot and I looked like a tray and pizza about ready to be shoved into the oven of this look-alike kitchen room.

If John and Hope hadn't sat there with me through this ordeal, constantly talking to me while I felt the alarming closeness of the equipment, and heard the weird clanks of the machinery, instead of focusing on the music that was piped in, I know I would not have been able to complete the test.

"Just keep your eyes closed I said," over and over again. "Pretend you are lying on the beach. Pretty soon it'll be over; you know you want the results."

A week later, I received the results from Dr. B and Dr. Chan. For all my heroic efforts, the MRI revealed a bulging disc on my left side. There were no images of my hips. Dr Chan still insisted that my leg problems were caused by a pinched nerve and that I needed to have X-rays of both hips and Dr. B suggested I see an orthopedic surgeon.

Taking another day off from school bothered me so much but it had to be done. An Amityville orthopedic surgeon, a member of my Empire Insurance Plan, was the next physician John drove me to see. My X-rays led to Dr. C's conclusion that I did, indeed, have arthritis in both hips, more as a result of walking on hard pavement than anything else. An anti-inflammatory was prescribed. In two weeks, he would see me again.

Lots of people had arthritis; in fact my good friend Penny had it in her hips for years; uncomfortable, surely, but life-threatening, no. I was relieved. Yet my pain increased, even with the medicine. Reaching out to Penny, she reassured me that I would learn to cope. Tina, a neighbor, who worked for an orthopedic surgeon, convinced me to get a second opinion. As fast as I could, I brought my images from one orthopedic office to another who took more X-rays of my pelvic region.

Listening to his diagnosis confused me: no arthritis, instead I had bursitis (in both hips), leg problems not related to my back.

What the hell was going on I wondered? Whom do I believe?

By the way he continued, I was to have more blood tests, including a test for Lyme disease. When both hips received a shot of steroids, I cried because I felt no pain. I cried from relief!

Following the doctor's advice I stayed home for a week, resting and coping with leg pains and twitches but no hip pain. My neighbor Maria drove me to get the next set of blood tests, for which I was so grateful. Her company helped me to stop dwelling on the thoughts that perhaps I had Lyme disease, something I knew little about, except that my sister's boyfriend had been diagnosed with Lyme and had been ill for a long time.

Continuing my chiropractic treatments with Dr. B, even though I knew he did not approve of the steroids, we did discuss the possibility of Lyme. Yes, he knew how tired I felt, but didn't blame that on stress, as I did.

When I found out that my blood test for Lyme was negative, I was thrilled. Yet, the question of neurological problems came to the fore; an MRI of my brain was ordered by the orthopedic surgeon. If there was any way to prolong this test, I was game. My job was suffering as much as I was, I felt, so waiting until the Easter vacation gave me the immediate out I emotionally needed. However, Marianne and Tina convinced me not to put it off.

Reluctantly I called Stony Brook for information about their Open MRI facility. A cancellation could secure my appointment that day; otherwise there was a 2-3 week wait. Something made me take the date.

Since I was shaken and too upset to tell my building principal; my good friend Katie took it upon herself to explain. I called John and Maria who drove me, along with my trusty bottle of wine, and of course, a paper cup.

John sat in the waiting room while Maria accompanied me to the "inner sanctum". The procedure was far easier, yet I kept my eyes closed and obeyed the orders not to move or speak. For an hour, Maria entertained me with her very welcomed chitter- chatter.

The results came in a few days; negative, thank God, ruling out Multiple Sclerosis. Although with the little I knew of this disease, I did not have the usual symptoms, except for the twitching and tingling which they said signified a neurological problem.

My friends and fellow teachers teased me when they heard my brain test was negative; "Nothing up there"! Joe, my principal laughed. "Oh, I knew it all along." Yes, we can find humor in almost about anything, I thought, but when I told Dr. B, he said he had heard of a case in which the MRI came back negative, but the patient still had MS.

Worry, relief, worry, relief, worry, re…………..When would it end? Where would it end!

Trying to hold down my job, the days were a struggle. One day a Special Delivery package was sent to me in my classroom. Opening it up in front of my excited students, we were all delighted to find a Vermont Teddy Bear, dressed in a hospital gown with a "boo-boo" bandage on its back and a note from darling Hope! A special gift since I "survived" the MRI! I quickly named him TR after Teddy Roosevelt, the president we were studying.

When TR came home I put him on the couch in the den and every time I saw him I recalled the MRI and what a dear friend I had in Hope; a perfect name for the sunny, cheerful girl who knew just how to brighten tough moments in my days!

Chapter 5

MUMBO JUMBO

About a week before the Easter vacation, each day became a dreadful struggle. Never in my life had I ever experienced such tiredness. A fairly good night sleep still left me fatigued during the day. It was like a damned if I do, damned if I don't game. Barely making it through each school day, I practically collapsed when I got home and could not cook, clean or shop. With just a week to go now, somehow my determination pushed me through.

During my appointment with Dr, B he mentioned, as a matter of fact, that I could have Chronic Fatigue. "What's that?" I asked.

"Epstein-Barr virus; another name for Chronic Fatigue," he said.

"You could take a blood test," he offered. "I'll wait," I replied, knowing he was leaving for a week vacation in Florida.

For some reason I started to clean or I should say, I tried to start to clean after I got home that day, found it impossible and became very distraught. I called Tina at the doctor's office to see what they thought about my extreme fatigue and if an Epstein-Barr virus blood test was needed. Tina explained the doctor seemed to know I would not be getting any better and a neurologist was the person to see. Back to this again! A Manhasset physician was recommended.

Following his advice, I called Dr. David Lang, and made an appointment for the day after Easter. I also notified Dr. B who said to me, "When are you going to call me with some good news?"

That Easter was the worst Easter of my life and I knew John felt the same. After Easter mass, we went for a ride to the beach where I told John I couldn't go with him to his Mom's for dinner and insisted he go without me. There is no doubt that I felt sorry, very sorry for myself, as I thought about so many past Easter holidays while I rested alone at home that afternoon. I wanted nothing to spoil the beautiful life John and I shared. Nothing made sense; nothing was in black and white. If I had not kept a journal I would not have been able to keep track of all that went on.

Monday morning arrived soon enough. What a way for John to begin his week's vacation. He and Hope drove me to Manhasset; no wine needed this trip. Arriving promptly at 9:00am we were greeted warmly by another short doctor who looked a lot like the actor Richard Dreyfuss. Highly recommended, very pleasant and professional, after looking at my rather thick folder, he agreed with the orthopedic's findings. After examining me and giving me a neurological exam, his diagnosis was vague; no real neurological disorder but "something" is going on. He further said my condition could be the beginning of "something" serious going on; it could stay like this or go away on its own and we'll never know what it is. So here I was hearing the words "something" and "it" but no words that pin pointed my condition. Flabbergasted, frustrated and furious described my reaction to what was a bunch of "mumbo jumbo".

What about MS? He didn't find anything specific to look into it, he told me. More tests would be expensive; it was up to me. If I couldn't return to school after this vacation, he felt it would cause me to sink to another level and offered Prozac to get me through, what he called "a stressful period". Recalling a Phil Donahue Show discussing the side effects of Prozac, I would be afraid to touch it.

What about debilitating fatigue? Is it possible I have the Epstein-Barr virus? His answer: "Why would you want that? There is no cure for that." I didn't want 'that' I wanted answers. Abruptly Dr. Lang stood and ushered me down the hall. "Where do I go from here?" my anguished voice pleaded. He thought for a half minute and told me I should have more testing done: blood work to test for a thyroid situation, an EMG, (electro myography) a nerve muscle exam.

Making my next appointment for Friday, before I left, and noting the charge of $300 for today's visit, and others to come, I thanked God for my insurance.

When I saw Dr. B the following day and told him what had happened with Dr. Lang, he felt hesitant to comment since he felt Dr Lang was in "another league", but expressed his relief that no neurological symptoms were seen. This very same day I pushed my way into getting an appointment with Dr. Chan. Desperation and impatience were my motives and after explaining what had transpired with Dr. Lang, I asked him to test me for Epstein-Barr virus. He agreed to do so and told me that I need not worry about MS at this time, but later down the line, I could be given a spinal tap.

Finally it was Friday! Once again John was with me for moral support which I really needed the moment we arrived. Evidently Dr. Lang was not the only neurologist here as I heard another physician trying to calm a woman who was in extreme pain. Obviously he didn't know what to do. I was so upset and nervous but picked up a People magazine for distraction, and by chance happened to see an ad for a TV series called "The Human Factor" with a photo of a kind looking gentleman smiling at me saying, "A doctor who gives; he thinks like a patient, acts like a doctor and feels just like you!" This is the doctor for me I thought, and I ripped out the page and put it in my pocketbook, to John's utter embarrassment.

At last Dr. Lang appeared, shook my hand, and led me to his office. Relating my yesterday's visit with Dr. Chan, a strange look came across his face; almost as if he was annoyed that I had seen Dr. Chan and even further put out that I was going to have an Epstein-Barr virus Test. If looks could kill, I would have been dead. Fortunately, I just walked away into his inner office for the EMG exam and continued talking. When I mentioned that I still had a tingling sensation in my feet along with a throbbing pulsation, he joked that maybe whatever this was would eventually leave me through my feet, and that he would attach the electrodes to my feet for the test. Strange behavior, for sure.

During the twenty minute test, I asked if this could determine whether or not I had MS, to which he replied that this was a nerve test and I was scoring better than any patient he had seen. "But let's wait to see what the blood test shows" he said. When I mentioned how exhausted I continually felt, and was sure it was something in my blood, he asked how I could possibly know the difference between fatigue and stress when doctors couldn't even tell the difference.

The tone in the room was almost offensive. Recommended or not, Dr. Lang made me feel very uncomfortable. We returned to his office where he recorded my results into his tape recorder. Again he offered to write a prescription for Prozac which I again declined. He asked for my work phone number and John's and said he would call next week with my results followed by another walk to the waiting room; another perfunctory handshake.

Returning to school on Monday and learning during my lunch break, when I called Dr. C, that I did have EBV gave me quite a sense of relief. I remembered 'everything is relative'; the diagnosis could have been far worse. I celebrated with hugs and kisses from the faculty! Dr. C didn't tell me to "take two aspirins and call me in the morning," but what he said was similar. "Just take some B vitamins with iron and if you don't feel better in a week, call me and I'll give you a B12 shot." Too tired and feeling almost defeated, I said nothing.

When I spoke to my friend Mindy (who had EBV) later that day, she verified that she, too, received the same advice from her doctor, and suggested I get the book titled, *Chronic Fatigue Syndrome*.

My next conversation was with Dr. B to report that I had EBV. Not an easy thing to live with, he claimed, but I was convinced I would do all I could to regain my health. That very evening, I convinced John to take me to the mall so I could purchase the vitamins and the book. As soon as I found the Chronic Fatigue book by Dr. Jim Stein I held on to it all the way home.

Would you believe I never received a call from Dr. Lang with his test results? I wanted to call him to tell him in no uncertain terms how unprofessional he was. Perhaps his ego was damaged when he found out that I had EBV and not some neurological illness. In any case, he was certainly not a credit to the medical field, and upon looking back I do wish I had "set him straight".

Chapter 6

WHAT ARE THE ODDS?

What are the odds you pick up a book, read it and the following week you have an opportunity to meet the author? Pretty slim, I'd say.

From the moment I began *Chronic Fatigue Syndrome*, I could not put it down. I felt this book was written just for me. Not only were all the symptoms I had been complaining about addressed by Dr. Jim Stein but his friend and physician, an "exceptional patient" Charles Peterson, had developed a "mysterious illness" who sought help from Dr. Stein who practiced non-traditional medical methods known as Alternative Medicine.

Stein discovered that Peterson had incredibly high levels (titers) of EBV along with a crippling form of arthritis. Using Charlie as a "guinea pig", as a way to bring his illness under control, Stein noted that his basic symptoms were severe pain and fatigue. In fact, Charlie was barely awake for more than a few hours a day.

Implementing homeopathic methods, Stein, a licensed homeopathic physician, treated patients with vitamin supplements in huge doses, and extracts of animals, vegetables and minerals in minute doses to help trigger the body's natural healing process. All of this was new to me; I had never heard the word homeopathy much less how to pronounce it! As I read each page, I could feel the beat of my heart, thumping and racing under my skin; a fortuitous celebration.

In his book, Dr. Stein outlined the specific protocol he used for Charlie as well as other patients during their long struggle. According to traditional medicine there is no cure for Chronic Fatigue. On the other hand, Stein actualizing alternative medicine, claimed to have developed one.

I couldn't wait to tell Dr. B about this book and what I learned. It became apparent that he, too, was excited and interested. I took my anxiousness a step further and said, "I'd even drink liquid heroine to get better," I admitted to him! In all reality, this was the time I felt that I would undoubtedly go through some very tough situations, but I knew whatever happened, I would be okay. Had God whispered to me?

And so it was as my physical health deteriorated and my emotional stability became more and more fragile, I blew up one day over a minor incident in my classroom. The shocking realization of my behavior led me to ask my principal for a week or two off from school. Sensing my pain, but knowing my love for my job and concern for my students, he tried to persuade me to stay; I left in the middle of that day.

One day the following week I purchased an updated version (the new edition) of Dr. Stein's book which described his practice in Great Barrington, Massachusetts and his new offices in Tuscon, Arizona. Telephone numbers were listed. Should I call, I wondered? After dialing a couple of the numbers and reaching answering machines, I gave up calling, but not losing my focus. All of a sudden I remembered Dr. B's receptionist Shari whose cousin had CFS so badly he had been bedridden for six months.

Through Shari a time was arranged for Barry to call me. "Did you ever read the CFS book by Jim Stein?" was the first thing Barry said when I answered the phone. My enthusiastic answer prompted him to say, "Would you open the book to the acknowledgements and read the first paragraph?"

It began with Stein expressing thanks for: "Vinnie Vita and Barry Clark for sharing in the dream of a comprehensive holistic health-care facility where the entirety of the treatments described within this book can fully manifest to offer hope and care to those who suffer or desire a higher quality of life."

"I am that Barry Clark," Shari's very friendly cousin told me. Feeling like I just received almost the best gift anyone could give me, I was so surprised and excited, that I could hardly wait to hear more about Barry and what he was going through.

Barry began by telling me how he'd been sick for about a year, how he made doctor's appointments after doctor's appointments, how he could no longer work and found himself relegated to his bed, thinking he was dying of some sort of cancer or Aids. Even in bed, he kept his vigil by asking his wife, Sue, to buy him book after book. By pure chance, like I did, he, too, found Dr. Jim Stein's "Bible".

Fortunately, Barry with the help of his wife, managed to endure the long trip to Great Barrington where he was to undergo a week's treatment of blood testing, nutritional seminars, and private consultations with a psychologist. Stein's holistic approach involved the whole person, not just the "disease", he explained.

After continuing Stein's treatment plan for six more weeks at home which included a special diet, a variety of vitamins and homeopathic medicines, Barry felt he was improving and soon returned to work. For me, Barry's story was just what I wanted and needed to hear. And when he offered to "make a few phone calls" on my behalf, I was stunned! In fact, he continued, "Jim will be staying at my home in Queens this weekend; how would you like to meet him?"

Oh my God! "Yes," I almost screamed! "Are you sure it's okay?" "It's fine Gail," he said with a smile in his voice that I could almost see, and gave me directions and an approximate time.

Talk about the "light in the tunnel" - when I hung up the phone, I said aloud, "I am going to be alright!"

On that bright, sunny Saturday morning, wearing my taupe slacks, white tee shirt, a turquoise linen blazer and tan shoes and bringing a gift for Barry, *The Juiceman's Power of Juicing* by Jay Kordich, John and I drove to Queens. What a great feeling it was to meet Barry, this gentle, caring person who took so much time to talk to me and to arrange today's meeting. When Dr. Jim Stein shook my hand, I responded warmly to this kind, gentle man in his mid-thirities who reminded me of a Teddy Bear!

I gladly answered Dr. Stein's series of questions regarding my symptoms and reminded him that my CFS didn't start with the flu to which he replied, "Not all cases do; however I would like to send you for a battery of blood tests at the National Health Lab in Plainview. We can review them in June when you will come to Great Barrington." "In June," I sputtered, "what will I do till June?" "Gail," he smiled, "you need to be home resting, no working, follow the diet in my book; organic foods, Gail, and I'll get you a list of vitamins you should be taking."

Jim Stein offered to autograph my book; John, my dear John, fetched it immediately from the car. How many times have I read his words, "To Gail - with Light and Love - JS"?

We all said our good-byes with handshakes and a special Jim Stein bear hug for me!

On the way home my mind was in a whirl. "Organic foods?" I said to John, "Now where in hell am I going to get them?" "There's a health food store called Sherry's Place in Babylon village and you know our neighbor grows organic vegetables. At least that's a start." "Pretty stupid if you ask me," I wisecracked, yet knowing underneath I would follow all Dr. Stein's recommendations. We stopped at Sherry's Place on the way home and discovered there was also a Sherry's Place - the Restaurant. Little did I know then, that this, was the first of many trips, I would make to both places.

Chapter 7
JUST DO IT

The following is an overview of the regime I set for myself to begin the road to my recovery.

STEP I. I called a New Jersey number to order the vitamins recommended by Dr Stein which is his formula known as either breakfast, lunch or dinner immune boosters. The dose was two at breakfast, one at lunch and two at dinner. Similar in their make-up, they consisted mostly of Vitamin C, Beta Carotene, Chinese Herbs and Echinacea. Flax seed oil, also on the list, to be either mixed in a salad or added to juice, was very difficult to swallow. Gagging, my throat felt as if it was closing with a knot forming in my stomach one hour after each dose. It tasted like motor oil but I was determined.

STEP II. There were at least a dozen prescriptions for my blood work. John and I drove together to the National Health Lab and when the technician saw the list, she looked at me rather nervously and asked, "What's wrong with you?" I explained that I had CFS and was under the care of a specialist. After checking each test in some sort of manual, she drew eleven vials of blood from my arm.

Hurrah, I did it, but I never looked at the needle!

STEP III. I reviewed Dr. Stein's diet plan in his book, trying to actually memorize it for all the unfamiliar meal planning and shopping I would be doing. My basic diet was to include mostly vegetables, some fruits, some grains, and either chicken, turkey or fish once a day. Red meats, fried foods, caffeine, and alcohol were to be eaten or drank in limited amounts but white flour and sugar were to be avoided. After following this simple, low-stress diet for the liver and immune system, for a week, one may begin the elimination diet by adding foods that you may have an allergy to; one food at a time. First, add citrus fruits for a few days. If tolerated, move on to corn-containing foods, then egg and wheat products, dairy foods, finally yeast products.

As you can imagine, this system was a totally new concept for me, a definite challenge that entailed a completely different way to grocery shop and to read product labels. Preparing and cooking meals to follow this plan were also out of the ordinary for me but I was resolute to do all that I could to improve my health. A new cookbook, *Italian Light Cooking*, by Marie Simmons, including some of Jim Stein's ideas in her recipes, became my cooking guide.

John didn't complain about "our" new diet, yet I'm sure he'd rather have had a juicy steak, French fries and ice cream instead of having to settle for a salad, lentil soup and fruit for dessert. If I were John, I bet I would have snuck into a steak house every so often and feasted on a prime T-Bone! How lucky I was to have John on board for the new and very different course that affected us both.

Dr. B and I would talk and laugh together about our juicers. When he first told me "I juiced", I laughed and when

I asked him about his weekend plans, he said he would be stopping on his way home to buy vegetables for his juice machine. "Is that what you do for fun?" I teased him.

Jay Kordich's emphasis on persistence in using the juicer, as a vital way in which to regain his health, inspired me, and even if I "juiced up", what I called the ugliest concoctions, such as ones with the horrendous flax seed oil, I knew I was doing the right thing.

As a big coffee and tea drinker who could no longer continue to drink about five cups daily as I had for thirty years, I foolishly stopped cold turkey. The excruciating headaches that resulted, I thought, were part of my illness, and not, as I discovered later on, a result of sudden and complete caffeine withdrawal!

STEP IV. No longer in the classroom, and staying home for the most part, relieved my anxiety. Worry-free rest and sleep, which my body so desperately needed, allowed me the luxury of real hope that I was surely on the right track in my healing process.

My "library" consisted of every book on CFS that I could get. Some were so frightening and very depressing. Literature from the Center of Disease Control in Charlotte, North Carolina, was even more alarming when referring to MS as an offshoot of CFS.

How fortunate to have friends "in sickness and in health". I thought that was just a husband mandate! Hope and Bea called regularly, Katie and Laurie, too. Listening patiently to my detailed explanations of my disease and all I was learning about it, these girls never wavered in their support. On the other hand, my mother who only read a part about stress, in the book I gave her, convinced herself and my father that if I would stop bringing stress upon myself, I'd be okay. Since I "didn't look sick" she said, it must be psychological, which only served to alienate us further.

Each week I called my school principal telling him I needed just another week but after a few more weeks of absence I did let him know I might not be back for the rest of the year. To use so many sick days was unheard of for me but I really didn't feel up to returning at that point.

STEP V. My preparations for Great Barrington on June 26th began in May when I received a large envelope of several forms to complete. My program would include a one hour consultation with Dr. Stein, a one hour consultation with Dr. Neil Owens, Orientation Nutritionist, and two one hour consultations with Dr. Jeff Ross, Clinical Psychologist. The cost of the program was $685.00.

Also enclosed were directions on keeping a food diary for five days which was to be mailed to Dr. Owens for a computer analysis that would yield an exact measure of the vitamins and minerals in my five day diet in order to determine and create a specific optimal nutritional program for me.

To complete the psychological history form, all important events in my life were to be listed chronologically, in the hopes that they might reveal a pattern for sickness and health. In addition, all my medical tests were to be submitted, as well as a one hour telephone conference, in which I would be asked detailed questions about my illness.

Included in the envelope were brochures of inns and hotels as well as restaurants. Since I was coming from quite a distance away and needed to make our reservations, the information and photos of the Bed and Breakfast, Little Manor, very close to the Solstice Clinic, caught my eye. Along with a full English breakfast and afternoon tea, the Victorian charm and personal dedication to comfort had me in a dither. I was psyched to go!

Chapter 8

THE VULTURE

During the weeks that seemed to drag, since I was so anxious to leave for Great Barrington, it became obvious that I definitely would not be returning to school for the rest of the year. Once a week I would see Dr. B., more for moral support than for chiropractic therapy. He felt that my being back in the classroom would be the best thing for me and was disappointed that I wasn't. Yet, he listened to me patiently as I reviewed literature I had read about CFS, quietly absorbed all my diet details and allowed himself to be my sounding board. To this day, I don't know how he put up with me.

The telephone calls, flowers and get well cards I appreciated so much even if they reinforced my medical plight and feelings of remorse for my unfulfilled school year.

One day, Jane, a friend from my childhood, and with whom I had been teaching but not in recent months, since she was reassigned to an another building, called to wish me well, and seemed genuinely concerned about my health, even so far as making offers to find out more about local doctors who might be able to help me.

As per usual, I talked about Dr. Stein, his book and program.

About a week before leaving for Great Barrington, Jane called again, to tell me that her sister, a nurse couldn't find any information on my Dr. Stein and questioned his legitimacy. Not to worry, I assured her. Then she probed me for more information about my health, suggesting that perhaps I might have lupus or MS. Very uneasy, I managed to end our conversation, and actually cried telling John what happened. Jane came very near to bursting my newly found bubble of hope, I believe.

Tim, my good school friend and social worker, called me a few days later and to this day regrets what he told me during our conversation. He overhead Jane telling the Assistant School Superintendent that she heard someone was on a sick leave and that she wanted the position in September. Shocked but on my toes, I asked him to repeat what he just said. "I'll f----- kill her," I yelled. How could she say that? I hadn't even thought that far!

Poor Tim; he was distraught, but interrupted my tirade long enough to add that the Assistant Superintendent replied, "Mrs. Wench is using her sick days. Her position is not available; she will be back in September." Begging me not to report this to Jane since it would implicate him, I promised I wouldn't, yet I called Tom back a few days later to tell him he was asking too much of me.

Eventually, I did tell my closest and dearest friends whom I knew I could trust. While waiting for Jane to call again, I planned how I would discredit her lethal friendship. She never called but made several inappropriate remarks to my friends asking why she hadn't heard from me and spent the rest of the school year trying to find out about my condition. Each time she ran into a brick wall.

When I confided in Dr. B. about "the Vulture" I also told him that I would be going back to school in the fall if he had to carry me. He smiled.

Chapter 9

AT LAST

GREAT BARRINGTON, MASSACHUSETTS

It was Thursday, June 25th, the last day of school for the students and teachers in Lindenhurst. For me, it meant the day before my long awaited trip to Great Barrington! As a celebration, Laurie, Hope, John and I had an early dinner at Sherry's Place and then returned to our house and sang and laughed along with Laurie as she played her keyboard piano. The girls made plans for their summer vacation while John and I were so glad to finally be heading north the next day.

My "mental alarm" woke me at 3:30 am, a half hour before our alarm clock. Taking quick showers, dressing in a flash, and gulping down smoothies, we were on the road in the dark heading toward my light at the end of the tunnel. Don Imus entertained us as we drove along, making great time, and even stopping at a diner for breakfast. We passed the inn where we would be staying that night; a big white Victorian house surrounded by beautiful gardens.

At 8:00am, we pulled into the parking lot of the clinic which looked like it been an old barn or maybe a house. It was very early but we decided to see if it was open. While a very pleasant, elderly woman greeted us at the front desk, Dr.

43

Jim Stein appeared and welcomed us graciously as I blurted out excitedly, "So, do you have my test results? What did they say?"

"Let's wait to discuss them at your appointment," Dr. Stein replied, and disappeared as quickly as he had appeared.

As we waited patiently, we learned that the elderly woman was, in fact, Dr. Stein's mother, and as we chatted, she talked about Barry Clark and was delighted I had met him, too. Two young women patients joined us followed by a young, short, thin, man who introduced himself as Dr. Ross and another nice looking man with dark hair and a beard who was the nutritionist. We three patients were given a folder full of literature on CFS and a detailed out line of the program.

As soon as Dr. Stein reappeared he called me first and asked if I wanted John to come also. "Oh no," I answered bravely, "John's heard plenty already!"

Leading me in to a small room where we both sat down, he seemed a little nervous as he placed the long pages of my results in front of him. When he began by saying something about high anti-myelin antibodies, I got nervous that fast since I recalled it had a connection with MS. In a small, shaky voice I said, "I think I need to get John," and ran down the hall, calling his name.

Dr. Stein repeated what he had told me and explained that since I had an elevated level of anti-myelin antibodies it could be an indication of something as in an "auto-immune disorder" which was not CFS. So, he further explained, "forget about the book, we'll concentrate on what I just told you. If it is left untreated, it could lead to more serious illnesses such as MS". And as almost an after thought, he mentioned that my blood work mimicked Lyme disease, to which I quickly said, "My Lyme test was negative." His next questions, "Do you have mercury fillings in your teeth? And have you had root canal?" really took me by surprise. When I finally mumbled "yes" to both, Dr. Stein pointed out that an auto immune disorder could be caused by toxins in the environment, or heavy metals. "However," he said, looking directly at me, "at this point it can be reversed."

"Did you hear that, Gail?" John smiled, "You're going to be okay!"

Dr. Stein probably will never forget the look of fear and anguish on my face that day just as I had never felt so frightened and helpless. My abundant knowledge of CFS, by this time, for all purposes was useless. Now I was deep into an area of which I knew nothing. Did I feel like a fish out of water? No, I felt like I was up a creek without a paddle. Didn't someone once say, "Mankind's worst enemy is fear of the unknown?"

After a minute or so, (I think John and Dr. Stein were talking) he handed me a cup for a urine sample and met me in another room to draw blood. A tiny red drop fell onto my light pink Liz Claiborne cotton slacks (that spot is still there - a horrible reminder). Neither of us spoke.

My next session with Dr. Owens, who insisted upon being called Neil, was short. In record time, Neil gave me a pad and pen, while he hastily told me to go back on the elimination diet and to follow it exactly. The list of vitamins I was to order, and to progressively add each day, would eventually amount to sixty per day. I was to keep a journal of my daily diet and how I felt each day. Neil would call me in two weeks. "Did I have any questions?" he asked, concluding our conference.

As soon as I met with Dr. Ross, I noticed the box of tissues on the table next to me. "Oh Lord, will he try to make me cry?"

The last thing I wanted to do or almost the last thing was to spill out my life story. What I really wanted to do was to run out of this place and never, ever see any of them again.

Instead, I sat calmly and talked openly about what Dr. Stein had said to me. My main concern was if I'd be well enough to return to school in September. During their lunch together, the three would discuss my case, Dr. Ross assured me. In a very nice, soft, mannerly way, he also asked me about my lifestyle and about my illness and seemed to have a good understanding of what was going on with me. The hour passed fairly quickly and when he opened the door, John was right there, waiting patiently to take me to lunch. The afternoon session would resume at 2:00pm with Dr. Ross who would advise me of the course to pursue.

I wanted to cry and leave but John kept the focus as he drove into the downtown section and found some Cheers look-alike restaurant that was recommended to us. The itsy-bitsy blood spot looked as big as a red balloon on my slacks, my appetite was zero, and my previous hopes and positive dreams of this day were crushed.

John suggested we window shop a little while waiting to return to the clinic hoping to avert my thoughts. I wasn't a very nice, amiable companion so we went back and waited.

Hoping to see Dr. Stein once more, to ask him about returning to teaching, I was very upset to learn he was booked solidly for the entire afternoon. John found a way in which to speak to him while I was in conference and his answer was, "We'll see."

Dr. Ross told me that even though Dr. Stein felt I should get total rest, knowing my active life style and mind, he felt some walking was fine. If I went to the beach, I must use total sun block, hat and umbrella, he further lectured. "How about

I get a mummy costume?" I almost yelled. Maybe I should get a gun and shoot myself; me sick like this and pale as a ghost all summer - no goddamn way!

Breathing techniques and relaxation through meditation and visualization were next on Dr. Ross' menu. By using some of these concepts on a tape he would make for me to play twice a day, they, would help me heal. With my eyes closed and listening to my breathing as he softly spoke, he helped me achieve a state of relaxation. He then asked me to visualize my body with a healthy, strong and impenetrable myelin sheath. Promising to call in a month, we shook hands, and I left to find John.

We drove slowly back to Littlejohn Manor. At one point, I said to John I didn't want to stay the night and wanted to go straight home. But stay we did, as almost an unconscious good decision, as the elixir after the horrible day.

Two "male angels" greeted us and knowing the reason for our stay, made us feel so comfortable and when they insisted on giving us the largest room, due to a cancellation, at no extra charge, we were very grateful. Practically collapsing on the king size bed, we lay there silently, holding hands for a very long time.

It was a Chinese Restaurant for us that night. Steamed vegetables and rice, even without soy sauce, was edible, but bland. At least John could order normally. Again, it was another quick meal before we returned to the inn directly, and decided to sit in the front parlor for a bit. Exhausted and drained, (I knew John had to be, too) I just wanted to sit and stare, but wouldn't you know, a guest sat down next to us, introduced herself and a conversation began. She, too, was here to see a doctor to decide whether to have risky surgery on her brain tumor or leave it alone. To live with it, she was exploring alternative medicine. Listening to her, I didn't feel as sorry for myself and once again recalled the adage, "Everything is Relative". We said our good nights and good lucks and went to our room.

I couldn't wait for morning to come; take a shower, get dressed, have an English breakfast and get the hell out of Great Barrington and that's exactly what we did!

Chapter 10

GRASPING AT STRAWS

Determined to conquer my vaguely diagnosed, mysterious illness, the summer of '92 loomed ahead. It seemed as if July and August would hold my destiny. The only path for me to follow was the direction I received from Jim Stein and his team. When I asked Dr. Stein if I should have a doctor on Long Island since he was so far away, his comment was to the effect that traditional doctors would probably give me steroids. So there I was with a stringent diet, tons of vitamins/minerals each day, a bunch of homeopathic "pillules", and, oh yes, limited walking and no concrete medical conclusions.

I decided I should talk to Dr. Chan again. John came with me and so did all my test results, along with literature about Dr. Stein and his book. Dr. Chan gave a cursory look at Stein's material and suggested after I explained my fear of MS that I see another neurologist. He also mentioned his patient with MS who was "going downhill rapidly". When I tried to show him Stein's treatment regime, he barked, "Gail, I have other patients to see."

Gathering up my literature, tests and book as quickly as I could, I walked out of his office. It would be the last time I saw Chan or any other traditional doctor for a long time.

49

As the days passed and I could barely manage the cooking and cleaning, the thoughts of finding help went against my years of self-imposed independence and only made matters worse. Some days I managed to drive to the beach and read parts of Dr. Ross' recommended book, *Minding the Body, Mending the Mind*, by Joan Borysenko, Phd.

As I read more and more, Dr. Borysenko's power of the mind to boost one's immune system and eventually overcome stress related, chronic pain, intrigued me and gave me the feeling that I had control of my illness. Norman Cousins' classic best seller, *Anatomy of an Illness*, supported Borysenko's theory that the mind was the key. An improved mental attitude for Cousins, however, was through comedy; good old-fashioned, belly laughing fun.

Next I read a book by Louise Hay, *You Can Heal Your Life*, who felt that we are responsible for our health; good or bad. Stuffed with so many theories, exercises, tapes, meditations, funny movies, comedy skits, soul searching and God knows what else, I was frustrated and confused. Yet, the one thing that did stick in my mind was Borysenko's definition of the term "peace of mind" To be totally immersed in whatever was happening at the moment, according to her, was peace of mind. "The most beautiful scene leaves you empty if your mind is full of worry," was one of the ways she brought this home to me.

Discussing some of my new findings long distance with Dr. Ross, I referred to my mental attitude when I was laid off from work the year before last. I remembered the "light bulb" which blinked, "Change the ways you look at things." If only I could do that now, I lamented. However, the big difference between then and now was the hourly reminder of how awful I felt. Dr. Ross would get a phrase in every now and then but I just continued rehashing. He did say I had the right idea when I told him the only thing that was getting me through all of this was my desire to get better. Under the circumstances, I was doing quite well mentally, he also offered. Amazingly, I realized after a few more of our rather one-sided conversations, that I was engaging in the same old chatter as I had done with Dr. B. I discontinued the phone calls.

Dr. Owens and I continued our telephone conversations for awhile. His requests were becoming more and more difficult. Spending sometimes in excess of $300 a month for vitamins and not feeling any better, when he suggested increasing certain oils, which only upset my stomach, there was no sense in talking any longer.

During one of my phone calls with Dr. Stein, he referred to one of my blood tests taken in Great Barrington as having mercury. A "holistic" dentist is someone you need to see about your mercury fillings, he explained, and told me to look in health store newspapers to find one. When I mentioned this to Dr. Owens during one of our last chats, he disagreed with his colleague Stein, and said, only as a last resort would he approve of such advice. Don't these guys work together? "Never mind about Neil," Jim almost shouted, "you better look into the mercury filling issue, Gail."

There was no doubt Dr. Jim Stein opened yet a new can of worms. Immediately calling Dr. B, he told me that what I needed was not a holistic dentist but rather an understanding one and gave me the phone number of his dentist who also happened to be Bea's also.

Before I contacted Dr. Barbara Sloan, I called my family dentist who stated emphatically the absurdity of such a remedy.

"Only 1% of the population is actually "allergic" to mercury," he confirmed and felt I was a very unlikely candidate. "Besides the AMA will not endorse this theory," he further educated me.

Yet I pushed on and made the call to Dr. Sloan. Intrigued and anxious to meet, her kind and sympathetic manner prompted my decision to see her as soon as possible. Although she was unfamiliar with the mercury-filling health relationship, she, too, sought alternative medicine when her illness, a few years ago, baffled traditional doctors.

My next call was to Barry to update him on my current situation. Ironically, Jim never advised Barry to have his fillings removed; a procedure Barry was almost ready to have done in Colorado by a a doctor and author of a book about mercury fillings. When he met Jim Stein, he decided against it. "Why don't you get that book, Gail," was all Barry had to say.

All the bookshops I called had never heard of the author or the book. I did find, *The Complete Guide to Mercury Toxicity from Mercury Fillings,* by Joseph Taylor, D.D.S. and, Guy Fasuina's, *Are Your Dental Fillings Poisoning You?* Devouring these books, I found what Jim Stein claimed: An illness such as CFS and/or an auto-immune disease *might* be cured by removing the fillings. However, there were no tests to definitely prove the patient's dental work was the cause.

Because you, my dear patient readers (no pun intended) must think I have really gone too close to the edge, please know that as a teacher, whenever I was asked a question to which I didn't know the answer, I would damn well find the answer. I trained my students to do the same. There's nothing wrong with not knowing but there sure is something very wrong when one doesn't take the steps to find out.

Because of the vague and ambivalent answers given to me from a field I had held in esteem, it became my job to search for correct information or as near to the plausible as I could find. The Diagnostic Center in Colorado would not recommend a dentist on Long Island until I promised to read the obscure book, they indeed had, and coerced me into purchasing one from them.

Waiting in Dr. Sloan's pink and gray waiting room with Stein's book, and all the information collected on the dental mercury issue, I had a good feeling of what was to happen here. From the moment we met, she put me at ease and was very willing to listen to me about a subject she knew little about. The time she took, and the encouragement and kindness she gave so graciously, I remember to this very day.

After reading most of the Colorado dental book, I called the Center again and was "rewarded" by the names of two Long Island dentists who were trained to follow the basic procedures in mercury amalgam removal.

Dr. Norman Browne, a holistic dentist in Nassau County happened to be the one Jim Stein suggested I find on my own. Again John came with me and we both noticed how much like a living room his office looked. Just as said in the book, no dentist will tell you that your illness is definitely due to mercury poisoning; Dr. Browne beat around the bush and advised I take a bio-compatibility blood test to find which type of composite fillings would be compatible with my body. The cost of removal of my fillings and replacement with a composite would cost approximately $3,500. He also suggested that my root canal be removed and replaced by a bridge, of course, for an additional fee.

When Jim Stein asked me what Dr. Browne "thought" I explained that he felt there was no way to find out whether or not mercury was the culprit. "Wait on this Gail; it's costly and chancy," Stein advised.

"Shit John," I screamed, "What do I do now?"

During this time frame, I had heard, as most everyone had, that Annette Funicello, who had been ill for quite awhile (with some symptoms similar to mine) had MS. Interestingly, she had sought some treatments in the Bahamas. Why hadn't she had her mercury fillings removed, I wondered?

My world had turned almost upside down. All this new stuff I was reading, and hearing, and listening to was either quackery, or could my illness be all in my head?

Chapter 11

THE THIEF OF TIME

By the end of July I somehow knew that returning to school in September would be out of the question. Could these thoughts have been with me since I told Barry Clark how worried I was about my job? Recalling his words, "Gail, this is not your way now, it is God's way. What will be may not be on your time schedule any longer," surely seemed prophetic. Coming from a man who had been so ill for two years, his view, however dim, was transparent.

Determined to keep the news secret until it was official, especially because of "The Vulture", I told only my closest school friends. My Department Chairman Jack, whom I trusted, advised me to discuss my situation, with our principal. Apparently understanding, he suggested I speak to the school physician, Dr. Gerome, and pointed out that I need not give any notice until a week before school began if I was not returning. How very relieved I was to hear his advice!

As usual, I brought my "stuff" to the appointment with Dr. Gerome, an allergist-immunologist, whose friendly smile and greeting when he'd pass my classroom, put me at ease immediately. Listening patiently, he seemed to understand my predicament and offered Lyme disease, MS and all the other as possible afflictions, I had already ruled out by test results.

55

56 | *Gail Wench*

Looking at me sadly and giving me a hasty exam, he found nothing wrong with my heartbeat and breathing but said my blood pressure was high. "Before all this," I said, "my pressure was on the low side," to which he replied, "Anyone going through what you have explained should have high blood pressure!" Concluding that I was probably "lucky" to have found Dr. Stein, he would write a letter to the school superintendent noting Stein's diagnosis and the treatment I was receiving.

Time has a way of fleeting by during good times and bad times and all too soon I found "time" running away from me. And so it was one morning in August when Laurie drove me to my principal's office for the appointment I dreaded. Joe Pisano and I spent an hour together. Knowing how much he believed in me, and assuring me my position would be there whenever I returned, he also promised not to divulge my circumstances until the last possible minute. When we shook hands, he saw the gratefulness and tears in my eyes.

A little smile crossed my lips as I walked back into the hall: no longer did I have to worry about "The Vulture"; Joe would see to that.

Wouldn't you know that when I was leaving the building, two of Jane's friends "pounced on me". "Are you coming back in September?" one asked. "Am planning on it," I said, smiling.

The week before school began without me, my Department Chairman, Jack, asked me to meet him for lunch. Reluctantly I agreed.

When I met Jack outside of the local Lindenhurst restaurant, he told me Joe and the assistant principals along with the secretaries were inside having lunch. "Oh God Jack, you don't expect me to go in there, do you?" "Gail, we have to; told them I was waiting for you."

After exchanging "hellos" we sat at a nearby table. Jack could see me trembling as I said to myself, "What are the chances that the superintendent will join them?" In a flash, he walked in, nodded to us, and sat down. Quietly, Jack tried to assure me everything would be alright. How could it be alright with a supposedly very sick teacher, who had a tan and was all dressed up, having lunch in a restaurant? Was I wrong to entertain a devastating premonition?

Chapter 12

MOUNTAIN CLIMBING

During Barry Clark's recuperation he heard a lecture by Dr. Goldman, a chiropractor, to whom, he later credited his "cure" along with Dr. Jim Stein. Encouraging me to make an appointment with Dr. Goldman, Barry tried to explain to "to my deaf ears" that unlike traditional chiropractors, he used a technique called "applied kinesiology". One chiropractor was enough for me. Dr. B fulfilled that role as well as the title "A Good Friend".

There were several lectures offered here and there but of no interest to me. Finally, I agreed to attend a Goldman lecture with my good neighbors Sandy and John. At the last minute I didn't think I would make it, as the overwhelming fatigue, almost conquered me, yet something again inside me gnawed, pushing beyond my limits.

Dr. Goldman's lecture was held in his office waiting room where about twenty seemingly healthy people gathered, and like me, who wore my madras plaid blazer, white tee shirt, white pants and a tan, were dressed appropriately. When a small, young, well-dressed man with a pleasant, yet serious demeanor entered the room and spoke, I was impressed by what I saw and heard.

"Everyone has Epstein-Barr virus by a certain age and if a doctor tells you that you have EBV, it simply means that your Epstein Barr level may be elevated for a variety of reasons," the young doctor began. Got my attention! But, before you learn my decision, here follows the essence of his lecture:

He explained that although one's Epstein Barr might be elevated, it is not considered a state of disease. Your immune system can be affected by the foods you eat, the water you drink, the lotions, gels and hairsprays you use and by the environment in which you live and work, he maintained. Certain foods may cause weakening of the immune system, just as the chemicals and metals in water can be damaging, and there may be toxins in the carpets we walk on, the paints on our walls and the mattresses upon which we sleep.

Without us even being aware of the toxins around us, until one day when our immune system decides it cannot handle all of the stress being put upon the body, do we experience physical symptoms. And if our immune system is compromised, Goldman went on to explain, both your adrenal glands and your thymus gland may be affected. Blood tests and "applied kinesiology" (muscle testing) can evaluate the condition of your immune system.

Offering to demonstrate how AK (applied kinesiology) works, he led us into another room and asked for a volunteer who was "healthy" and one who was "ill". Preferring men because they are generally stronger, Goldman explained that he would use the leg and arm muscles of each man to test for strength. All of a sudden the quiet group stirred and whispers, deciding who would be the two guinea pigs, buzzed around the room. I'm glad John didn't offer, as I wanted him right next to me; the healthy husband of the woman sitting to my left volunteered.

Each would have to hold up one leg or arm in the air and try to resist the pressure that he (Goldman) would create by pushing down on either limb, the doctor explained, noting that most people can keep their arm or leg in position, which they did. But when the doctor directed the "ill" man to place his hand over his adrenal or thymus gland and try to resist with his other arm, his arm became immediately weak. Embarrassed that he couldn't resist the pressure as he did with the first test, Goldman nodded, smiled and said, "You were perfect; you did just what you were supposed to do."

Because an ill person's glands do not work efficiently, the results of the test we witnessed were expected. To treat this problem, Goldman prescribed vitamins, herbs and other homeopathic remedies. It seemed to me like a game of give and take; give the body what it needs and take away what it doesn't need; simple!

The skeptical walked out; most stayed. None of what transpired seemed harmful to me and since Barry Clark had sung his praises, and the fact that I was running out of time, for all practical reasons, including the miracle for which I constantly prayed, I made an appointment with Dr. Goldman for the following week.

Clutching a new set of straws, I gradually dropped Stein's program, dared Dr. Goldman to prove to me that I could get better, and secretly knew I would go to any length, even a "far-out" method, ignoring any criticisms.

Indeed I knew it all sounded crazy, but I was desperate, and so twice a week, Tuesday and Thursday evenings I met with Dr. Goldman. He would "muscle test" me, using the various items I brought, such as the water I drank, commons foods I ate and my body products.

At the onset, he felt I was testing very strongly for the person I claimed to be! All my "items" were fine except for my body substances. Sherry's Place Health Food Shop fulfilled my need to purchase natural equivalent products. Soon these, too, tested "strong".

Now what do I do, I wondered? To me I was the rock in a hard spot. By the process of elimination, Goldman resorted to his fourth and last test. Something in my home might be the problem, he suggested, and wanted to examine my environment, of course for a fee ($150). But first, he asked me for samples of my carpet and hall wall paint. I decided to bring in a sample of our mattress, too, much to John's chagrin, but the mattress was old and nothing would stop me.

Like the final setting of a murder mystery when all is quiet, with many pairs of eyes focused upon the item being tested and nerves of steel riveted to the outcome which would reveal the link between the killer and the object, the night of the test, I walked in slowly, grasping the shredded piece of mattress in my hand as if it were the most valuable object in the world. Holding on as tightly as I could to that ripped fabric, while Dr. Goldman performed the test, my eyes and ears were at peak attention. The results were "WEAK" to my grateful joy. AH - HA, the mattress must go tomorrow; no, TONIGHT!

My excitement, my jubilation, were short-lived when Dr. Goldman said if I were really interested in getting a new mattress, I would have to wait until I found one that was suitable, so that when he tested me again, I would test "strong". To my amazement, he offered to meet me at a mattress store in Commack to test me on them!! Yes, you read correctly, this was exactly what he said. To boot, he would not charge me for the time this would take.

The following afternoon, Hope and I drove to "One Stop Sleep Shop" in Commack and waited for Goldman to meet us. After arriving much later, due to heavy traffic on the L.I.E., we entered the store. At once a salesman recognized Dr. Goldman. Together the three of us went from mattress to mattress, "muscle testing" as we went along. When I saw a Serta Perfect Sleeper that happened to be on sale, I prayed for the correct test result. Happily, I tested "strong". Goldman tried to lower the price even further, but the salesman wouldn't budge and because it was the only one left, a re-order would take at least a week. I agreed to take the mattress "as is".

Before he left, Dr. Goldman told me he would be at my house the next day to complete the testing. While Hope and I sat with the salesman as he wrote up my bill, he told us that the doctor had been in the shop from time to time with other patients and at first he (the salesman) thought "he was fuckin' nuts" but had learned that more than one person claimed the doctor cured them. Never once had Goldman asked for a cut or referral fee which I was very glad to hear.

When I asked our friendly salesman if the mattress could be delivered the following day, he said it would take a week! Wait till John hears this, I said to myself. We had been sleeping on the sectional in the den since I told John to throw out our mattress the day before yesterday.

They say you have to climb the mountain before you can see the view. I felt as if I was finally near the very top!

Chapter 13

FOURTEEN DOORS AND A MATTRESS

Dr. Goldman, his wife and two daughters arrived on Saturday afternoon. After we all greeted each other, the doctor and I got down to work. Either touching an item or lying down on it while Goldman "tested", I was very glad when the carpeting passed the exam! The paint tested "strong", too. Traipsing through the house the only detrimental objects he could find, besides the mattress which was already in the garage awaiting pick-up, were the fourteen doors. Because they were stained, a shellac would most likely do the trick, the doctor advised.

"Without your fourteen doors and a mattress Gail, you should be feeling a lot better in a few days," grinned Goldman.

Remember when I was told to watch comedy shows? Well, now here I was co-starring in one of the most ridiculous shows I could imagine. But we needed a new mattress and who cared what the doors looked like anyway, I had to get better!

Pocketing his fee, Dr. Goldman left with his family in tow, reminding me of my Tuesday appointment.

Our friend and neighbor, "Pete the Painter" who painted our house when we built it six years ago, would be happy to help us again I knew, and he came right over after I called

65

him. Not only would he shellac the fourteen doors but he offered to lend us his air mattress until our new one arrived. Not once did Pete ask why I was sick or question the work involved; he was just anxious to help.

By that evening the fourteen doors were in the garage awaiting "their treatment" and the air mattress, with a slow leak, was set up on the hardwood floor. Laughing together during the night as the mattress gave way, I couldn't help but think that I must be a little crazy to go to these lengths to try and regain my health.

As the days passed, much as they had previously, I continued to bring various articles to Dr. Goldman for testing. My twice a week appointments helped our doctor patient relationship but I knew I wasn't any better. When friends told me to drop him like a hot potato, I shrugged off all negativity.

I also kept seeing Dr. B regularly but kept mum about my latest guru, afraid he would be insulted. However, one day as luck would have it, when I mentioned something about my filtered water being tested he asked where I had it tested. Reluctantly, I told him about Dr. Goldman. The look on his face as he stated what Goldman was practicing was not legitimate, nor was his diagnosis, clearly indicated his disgust. Begging him to stand by me, and continue to help me for I was doing everything I could do to get well, even participating in Goldman's methods which I believed weren't harmful, he grudgingly agreed.

Meanwhile, Jim Stein assured me if Dr. Goldman's treatment didn't help; he had some other plans in mind for me. And so it was, in one last ditch effort, Dr. Goldman thought I might have Lyme disease, since there was "something" he said, trapped in the muscles in my legs. He sent me to Stony

Brook Hospital where I prayed for a positive diagnosis so that a treatment and cure would follow.

It wasn't long before the negative test results came back. My tears along with Goldman's disappointment could not change the facts. Now it would be back to Dr. Stein for me I told him, and I also mentioned a book that I had just read, by a renowned Manhattan doctor. Immediately Dr. Goldman recalled some of his patients who had been to Dr. Adams in Manhattan and came to him afterwards. Adams' treatments for CFS did not work for them; nor would they for me.

Jim Stein began some new treatments with me. Prescribing a ten day course of tetracycline with the provision that homeopathic injections three times a week instead of the weaker pillules, would be ordered if the tetracycline didn't help, became the next regime.

Ten days later I ordered the injections. Barry Clark had sworn by them. Willing but not able, since I could not inject myself, I couldn't ask John to do what I wouldn't do and I wouldn't think of asking a friend. Mentioning my predicament to Dr. B and Shari (she and I were good friends by this time) they both offered to do it! Guardian angels seemed to always appear when I most needed them.

Dr. Adams' book intrigued me and when John told me that one of his employees had been to the Adams Center for Complementary Medicine in Manhattan and "swore by him" I contacted her. Happy, as she was nicknamed, had hypoglycemia, and had felt tired and sluggish for a long time. Spending time with me over the phone, Happy told me many things about his program, especially his nutritional approach to good health and recommended his radio show at 9:00pm on weekdays. The Adams newsletter she sent me,

I showed to Dr. Goldman to no avail. He was firm in his beliefs.

Not to be deterred, I would still give Adams a try, although my intent was a lot easier said than done. Little did I know that the worst was yet to come.

Chapter 14

MOVIN' ON

Happy's copy of Dr. Adams' newsletter on CFS became my bible. After reading it at least thirty times I was very familiar with what he thought were the causes of CFS as well as his intense regime for a cure. Diet and vitamins coupled with vitamin drips as well as removing silver/mercury dental fillings were the treatments he advocated. Since Adams was a medical doctor as well a nutritionist, with world wide recognition, I made an appointment at the Adams Center for testing on Wednesday, November 11th (Veteran's Day).

Arriving at the center an hour early, John and I were impressed by the swanky lobby where we waited which was part of the six story brownstone that had been remodeled. Grays, blues and greens were the main colors within this ultra modern building. Treated extremely professionally from the onset, I felt good about the decision I had made.

Six vials of blood were taken, then seven more for the Glucose Tolerance Test. A physical exam, a psychological exam and interview, a urinalysis, a cytotoxic food allergy test, a live cell analysis, a mineral analysis and other basic lab work were also performed, all in clock work order.

We were both famished by the time we left, but drove straight home, stopping at Sherry's Place, to sit quietly while

69

we stuffed our faces! My state of catharsis from the day's events kept me upbeat as did Adams' book, newsletters and his nightly radio show. Now I wanted to meet the man.

Due to a cancellation, I was given an appointment on the Monday of Thanksgiving week at 4:00pm, otherwise it would be a six week wait. Although the time was very late, we both jumped at this opportunity, but I prayed that I would be alright since a long day sometimes would just wipe me out.

While we waited that afternoon, we saw Dr. Adams as he came out of his office, glance around and call his next patient. I asked John what his initial reaction was to the doctor; John didn't like him, neither did I.

When he came out for me and my folder, he looked at the test results and the twenty or so pages I had copied for him, obviously for the very first time. All of a sudden looking up, he asked, "Oh, this CFS, it came on all at once?" I replied, "If it is CFS, I'm not certain of anything at this time." Although he suspected Lyme or MS, there wasn't enough evidence to evaluate that either, he stated, and, like Jim Stein, he labeled "it" CFS and an auto-immune illness, but added that I also had hyperglycemia and candida. His instructions were to follow his diet and vitamin plan along with several IV vitamin drips. My fillings must be removed and my root canal removed, followed by IV Chelation Therapy for each removal.

Next, his nasty little nutritionist reviewed a very restricted version of the Adams' meat and mullet diet. He also informed me of the fact that after spending $100 on vitamins, I would receive a copy of Adams' Health Revolution. I could foresee lots of his books to wrap as presents.

Once more John and I hurried home, stopping at the Beachtree Café, near our house for a late dinner.

Of course I wanted to tell Dr. B what had occurred with "the man himself". "I'll fucking starve to death on this diet," I told him as he read the sparse offerings, while I described Adams as a "pompous ass" and quickly added it was his knowledge I was paying for, not his personality. The low-carb, high protein diet consisted of meat, eggs, vegetables, very few grains, no fruit, sugar or yeast and eggs and heavy cream as far as dairy. That was it. But instead of waiting "to starve to death on the diet", I "would die trying".

During the first week of the herald nutritional diet, I developed what is called "ketosis" which is a name for burning your baby fat. Fearing a weight loss, I decided to eat potatoes to maintain some substance.

The trips into Manhattan were grueling. John didn't just drive me because I wanted his company; he had to for I was too sick to drive myself. Taking a half day from work on Wednesday to drive me was the easiest for him; Saturdays he was off.

And so began the ritual which took me to the 3rd floor of the Adams Center, strictly for the IV patients, which reeked of vitamins and urine. Most of the approximately twenty five "victims" were much older than I and suffered from heart disease, cancer or aids. Often I would strike up a conversation with someone next to me to help the time pass faster. Dear John, who hated this as much as I, would often talk to the staff and even the patients, to help wile away the time.

One day we both started chatting with a friendly older woman called Catherine who was an ex-nun and ex-teacher but who now worked in a Queen's federal office building. She had lung cancer and refused chemotherapy and/or radiation. Her alternative regime was much more strenuous than mine and I marveled at her strength and will to continue. Working full time, she came here several times a week, all on her own! Looking at my dearest John, I thanked God again for him.

As I had mentioned, the staff here was wonderful but Clara who worked the IV floor, was absolutely outstanding. Her training as a Russian orthopedic surgeon put her in a category of her own. The special attention she gave to everyone was well appreciated and I was no exception. It was because of Clara that I began to accept this time as a different stage in my life and instead of trying to turn the tables to my advantage, I played with the cards I was dealt.

It was almost as if I was changing the way I looked at some things the day John and I brought in our favorite Seinfeld tapes. All of us: the patients, as well as the staff, had so much fun and laughed and laughed. What a change in our atmosphere that day!

Just before Christmas while I was getting my IV treatment, and watching a Neil Diamond Special on the TV, my surroundings looked so festive and there was a definite feeling of Christmas at the Center, where big, beautiful poinsettia plants decorated all the rooms. Yet outside, each day seemed gray and dreary, reminding me of some of the patients whose faces wore such sad, tired and worried expressions, except for that day in December when I thought I saw a glimmer of hope.

Chapter 15

HEAD CASE

Before I decided to leave Goldman and go to Adams, I had already made an appointment to see the holistic dentist Dr. Horrace Browne again. Bare with me, if you will, while I back track to that appointment.

John and I arrived at Dr. Browne's office on Halloween. Not only was the staff in full costume, he was, too! The big footed, red wigged, fat clown ushered us into his back living room/office where we talked about the procedure I would undergo. My concerns and questions out performed anything the clown might have had in mind and before we left, five appointments were on the books for Gail Wench, beginning the week before Thanksgiving.

If you can picture every bit of dental work you've ever had done in your entire life crammed into two hours, you understand what my first go round in that chair entailed. How I endured that session and the four that ensued is beyond description, just as is the fact that I even went when I felt utterly ill. After each torture session of needles, fingers, machines and tools accosting my mouth and teeth, when the Novocain wore off, the aching pain lasted for 24 hours.

Listening to a tape Dr. Browne had loaned me on the dangers of mercury fillings gave me some encouragement. At least I knew I wasn't insane to have agreed to the procedure that I prayed to God would work for me and cure what seemed to be my endless suffering. The mercury button he gave me with the slash through the mercury symbol, like the one he wore, I hid at home.

Only by God's grace could I ever have withstood the dental work and the Adams treatment at the same time. When John took me on December 18th to the oral surgeon to remove my root canal, the surgeon, who was not a firm believer in this method, took an X-ray and found an infection under the root. Could this have been the very cause of the breakdown of my immune system I wondered? After completing this last procedure, I was dismissed with a gauze-filled bloody mouth and a swollen cheek.

While John attended his Christmas work party that evening, I rested in bed, thanking God and praying again that I was along the road to where there was a light at the end of the tunnel.

Chapter 16

MY TWELVE DAYS OF CHRISTMAS

I have a pretty good idea about what all of you are thinking about right now. If she is so sick and exhausted all the time, how is she able to go to so many appointments and participate at the Adams Center? All I can tell you is that something led me not to give up. I would have rather died.

During my darkest hours with my circumstances almost too much to bear, there always were two choices. I could either prepare to expire or prepare to heal. Since I have always been a chicken, I knew I had no other choice but to battle for a better life. At least my good sense told me I wasn't alone for everyone has something they do not like; an obvious affliction, an invisible illness or even a bad habit. It seemed to me that either that which is hated remains to destroy or is changed for the better.

Indeed, just my one week schedule was incredibly demanding:

Saturday - Atkins IV Drip, Monday - Dr. Jim Stein staff appointment, Tuesday - Dr. B appointment, Wednesday - Adams IV Drip, Thursday - free, Friday - Root Canal, Saturday - Adams IV Drip, Sunday - free.

One day just before Christmas I wrote this "SONG" to describe my routine:

GAIL'S 12 DAYS OF CHRISTMAS

On the 1st day of Xmas my disease gave to me,
Vitamins in an IV.
On the second day of Xmas my doctors gave to me,
Two homeopathic injections.
On the third day if Xmas my dentist gave to me,
Three temporary crowns.
On the fourth day of Xmas my doctors gave to me,
Four chiropathic adjustments.
On the fifth day of Xmas my doctors gave to me,
Five bills of lading.
On the sixth day of Xmas my doctors gave to me,
Six eggs a-weekly.
On the 7th day of Xmas my doctors gave to me,
Seven Arizona phone calls.
On the 8th day of Xmas my doctors gave to me,
Eight teeth a-hurting.
On the 9th day of Xmas my doctors gave to me,
Nine more appointments.
On the 10th day of Xmas my doctors gave to me,
Ten vitamin bottles.
On the 11th day of Xmas my doctors gave to me,
11 drops of Echinacea.
On the 12th day of Xmas my doctors gave to me,
12 mercury free fillings.
BUT all I really wanted was my health back!

At this point I knew I had taken on too much. The demands of the schedule and procedures prevented my getting the rest needed. After Christmas, (with the dental work completed) Karen Paris, Dr. Adams' assistant, felt I needed just one IV each week instead of two. However, she wanted me to see an osteopath in Glen Cove to try some cranio-sacral therapy. Another doctor, another new face, another diagnosis, another treatment, another pipe dream..........

Chapter 17

DOCTOR GORGEOUS

Dr. Adams' assistant advised me that several of her patients had improved with the help of Cranio-Sacral Therapy and certainly I might, too, if I took the opportunity of five to six sessions. In the meantime, it would be wise to stop my chiropractic visits, which, of course, Dr. B would understand, but again his opinions, support and friendship were of great value to me. Phone conversations would have to do for awhile since I couldn't afford to leave even one stone unturned.

I was surprised that Dr. Marconi answered the phone when I called for an appointment. Maybe he was a one-man operation. In a young and very pleasant sounding voice he explained that he would not treat me until I read some literature on cranio-sacral that he would send me. Knowing absolutely nothing about the subject, I thanked him quickly.

The pamphlet that arrived reviewed the history of Osteopathy in the cranial field and described a constant movement inside the body of spinal fluid within the brain and spinal cord that can be felt with trained hands. As an involuntary, rhythmic motion, it transmits the rhythmic motions of the brain and spinal fluid through the membranes of the skull and to all tissues of the entire body.

I learned that the skull is not a rigid solid bone but rather separate bones that allow light movement. Moving these parts can somehow awaken the "patient within" to restore balance and harmony to the body. Evidently, the science of Osteopathy states that the body, if adequately nourished, can function to maintain, repair and heal itself.

None of what I read sounded dangerous or painful. I made the appointment. My dear friend Laurie drove me to Dr. Marconi's address where a very gracious woman greeted us in a second floor office, which was very small and very hot. In a few minutes, a tall, thin, young and good-looking man greeted us. Introductions were made while Laurie and I could just about hold our thoughts. Dr. Marconi was one gorgeous hunk!

Ready to examine me since I had reviewed a lot of my problems and symptoms when we talked on the phone, I took off my shoes, lied down on the table, and after a not so routine exam, he turned on some "new age" music and touched different parts of my body, listening to the motion of my spinal fluid. The touching and holding went on for about an hour and as I glanced at a painting of a sunset on the ceiling, I felt relaxed and quite peaceful.

I was to call Dr. Marconi the next day to report how I was doing and to make a follow-up appointment in a week. You probably can imagine how Laurie and I talked about the doctor's good looks on the way home.

Continuing for five weeks, I had hoped that something as simple and "crazy" like this treatment would work. No such luck, and by the end of treatment #5, there wasn't even the slightest iota of improvement.

And so 1992 came to an end, the year I call the most terrifying year in my life. How would this all end? What would 1993 bring?

Chapter 18

THE MASK

If I didn't look like "the type" to be sick, I was glad it wasn't visible. Truthfully, I was secretly proud and amazed when so many said, "You don't look sick." Psychologically, it was vital for me to "look good" and I did everything I was capable of doing to camouflage my illness. "Vanity, thy name is Gail" would be a good title for my obsession.

Keeping up appearances, I continued to do my hair, put on a little extra make-up, especially around my eyes, and dressed well. I could fool a lot of people most of the time, definitely in the morning when I was freshly "done up" but as the day wore on, so did I.

My vanity was the reason I got into a big argument with Dr. B one day as he never really understood how sick I was and often would continue prodding me to return to work. If he knew how badly I wanted to be at school, why did he constantly urge me to do what he should have known I couldn't do? He was as well aware as I was that my illness didn't even have a name, but that did not mean I was well. There were those who had cancer or aids, who could go to work each day and lead semi-normal lives, because the treatment they were getting allowed them to function. What, in hell, did I have that prevented me from functioning? An illness that was not defined, coupled with my "looking good", didn't exude sympathy from Dr. B.

And so it was that one day in January when I asked Dr. B. for the 100th time what my illness could be, he mentioned a few things again and then said he hadn't ruled out psychological causes. Shocked, I left his office in tears.

No matter what I pursued, not matter how I tried to look like a human being so I wouldn't become a burden on anyone, no matter what I tried to express to all the doctors, especially Dr. B it all seemed so useless. There was no "light at the end of the tunnel" but rather a deep, dark mass of contradictions. It was as if there was no way out.

Like a dog with a bone, I went back to Dr. B, this time armed with a book about CFS, in which I had underlined photographs of those afflicted with the disease and how they appeared "normal". Nevertheless, he still held on to his ideas, but in a friendly way.

Maybe I should have told him how I felt the day I left the dentist's office with my mouth numb and distorted from a long session when I stopped for a light, and some guy pulled right up next to me, beeped his horn, and stared at me. Some guys must be desperate, I laughed to myself. He saw a blond in a Camaro. I saw a woman with a mouthful of pain.

John was the one I could never fool. Just one look into my eyes was all he needed to know what kind of a day I was having. When he saw the dark circles under my eyes, before I put on my make-up, or late in the day, he was very upset.

A few of my friends tell me now, how they never wanted to let me know how sick I looked. And for that I am so grateful, for my self-consciousness and pride kept me from ever willingly letting down my guard.

Regardless of how I looked, I wasn't feeling any better. Worry and fear would almost overtake me and one morning when I allowed myself to think for too long, I thought I just couldn't continue this struggle with my body any longer and would have to succumb to give up. Miraculously, I did not surrender.

Chapter 19

ON THE BRIGHTER SIDE

Speaking to God was something I did every single day and asked him if there was a purpose to all of this. Was there some sort of substance to this that I was to learn? If I had the energy, I would have screamed my very loudest, "Enough already!" When I began to question my existence too frequently, somehow I realized that there was so much for which to be grateful.

First of all it was sunny days. Even in the winter, to wake up to sunlight was so uplifting. Sitting in my den during the day, feeling the warm sun on my face, was heavenly. Our beautiful home, our castle, which we had built seven years ago, an open, light, uncomplicated contemporary-colonial became my haven to gather my strength. It was my quiet place of refuge where I sat and read or rested or stared out of the many windows during the day or watched the flickering candlelight dance across the walls in the evening.

Sherry's Place, where so many of my necessities were purchased, and her restaurant, so quiet and peaceful, perched next to the canal, gave John and me many good meals in cozy surroundings. A new shop, the Beggar's Banquet, close to home, became almost a daily destination for me in late August when I went to the beach as much as I could and would order a salad and ice tea to take with me. Even when I was quite ill and canceled appointments, I would find a way to go there even for just a cappuccino, and visit with the owners, Joanne and Kevin. "When I get better," I told them one day, "I'm definitely giving myself a big party and you are going to cater it for me." Cheering, they happily agreed!

When the extremely inexpensive nail salon, Charming Nails, opened that fall, I made an appointment. Operated by Koreans who spoke very little English, they were perfection professionals, who pampered me so much that I could relax and find peace. Here was another place I gladly became a regular. Years later when the shop's new owners, Lisa and Andrew's beautiful renovation helped earn its new name Escape, because of the exquisite décor, music and top of the line spa treatments, it became an even more necessary and delightful refuge for me.

Although I had to give up walking during different phases of my illness, not walking at all made really no difference in how I felt. To become weaker by not walking at all was absurd and so I walked as much as I could.

Plants and flowers, oh, how much I enjoyed them. Treating myself once a week to a bouquet of fresh, delicate, gorgeous flowers just made me smile. If I were an artist I would have gladly painted their images all day long.

When I was teaching I would tape the Phil Donahue Show and the soap, Santa Barbara, watching them faithfully each evening. Now that I was mostly house-bound, I could watch them during their regular schedule. My life was very different; time almost stood still. All that I had previously juggled on weekends could be accomplished during an entire week if I was up to it.

Watching the "Good Day New York" show in bed each morning helped to control my thoughts that something awful was going to happen. Frustrated and debilitated as I was, the news staff, so upbeat and alive, sent welcomed signals to me. Their enthusiasm for life was often contagious. And, of course, John and I adored Seinfeld. He was a godsend and I became the ultimate Jerry Seinfeld fan!

Every Tuesday, 10:30am, like clockwork, I was there. How often Dr. B. listened to the latest episode of "my journey back to health" most of which he did not agree. Nevertheless he continued to befriend me. I was the patient; he was patient.

Every now and then I would add extra burdens to my already worrisome mind. How, I wondered, could John continue to find me attractive and want to make love? Yet, my illness had drawn us even closer together. How miraculous it was to be able to continue our lovemaking. My sense of myself as a woman who was desired by her husband kept my femininity visible and amazingly active during a time when I questioned everything.

Chapter 20

ENOUGH IS ENOUGH

Everyday while praying to God I would ask for my old life back. How I longed for my beautiful, simple, happy and productive life. But after a year with no improvement, I began to positively despair, and had decided that I would never be the same person I had been before this illness. In fact, my life would be changed forever.

Dwelling for days on my self-inflicted miserable thoughts, I changed gears, so to speak, and started to pray for my health. Asking for my old life was out of the question for it had finally dawned on me that I had already changed, and to go on in a better state of health was a far more realistic quest. And so my prayer each day asked God to show me the way to make myself better.

During one of my off and on conversations, during this time with Jim Stein, who seemed definitely frustrated with my condition, he asked when I had my last Lyme Test and suggested I have another urine test. When I replied that a recent blood test came up negative again, he didn't push it. But that night in bed I lay there thinking about it.

"Forget it Gail," John, said, "You don't have Lyme!" "All I have to do is pee in a cup, John, so why not? You know I don't want to take any chances."

The next morning couldn't come fast enough. Barry was my first call, then Jim Stein. A girl called Dawn would be calling me with the information I needed to take the Urine Antigen Test. In three days I received a box in the mail with the instructions to take a sample for three consecutive days. The first sample was to be taken as soon as I awoke and it had to be placed in the freezer; second and third days the same procedure. After the third day, I was to bring the frozen samples to the National Health Lab in Plainview where they would be sent on for further testing, before notifying me in a few weeks.

Chapter 21

MIXED EMOTIONS

A new president was elected. Today is Bill Clinton's Inauguration. I have been sick for one year. The line that keeps beating in my brain is, "I am out on a limb with a quack from Arizona."

Traveling to Manhattan once a week to the Adams Center was as routine as my constant fatigue. Two women patients with CFS/Lyme disease told me they had been sick for years and were no better with Dr. Adams. When I met with his assistant that afternoon and explained to her the Lyme-urine test I had taken under Dr. Stein, she was concerned, and suggested if there was no improvement by April to see a neurologist for a MRI.

At another crossroads, I debated whether I should drop Adams, stay with Stein and wait for the urine test report. Back and forth I went, as John, focused on the long ride home, listening to my dilemma. We stopped at the Parkwood Café in West Islip, our "ride home" favorite place for dinner.

On February 12th (Lincoln's birthday) Jim Stein announced to me over the phone, at 5:00pm, that my urine test showed high levels of Lyme disease. At least now there was a definite answer for my condition. Stating that I would now have to decide whether I would continue with him or go to a Long Island doctor, Stein sounded a little guilty but said "You've jumped around from doctor to doctor, Gail." To me that meant if I had remained with him solely he MIGHT have found this out sooner.

Wasn't he aware of the fact that I lost one year of my life due to incorrect test results, contradicting opinions and all sorts of other gross errors? Needing time to make a correct decision, I got off the phone, and called Barry, Bea and Laurie. Before the week was over I began my research of Lyme with a library book, and cancelled all appointments with Adams.

My new mission included calling all my former doctors. Some told me more tests were needed because the urine test was not reliable. When I called the Home Care Service they gave the names of three doctors on Long Island. Yet, I leaned toward Jim; he had to be involved. Naturally, my mother called to tell me of her lack of faith in Dr. Stein and suggested I get a second opinion.

Here I was using an alternative doctor who was now suggesting traditional medicine, unknown to me, in extreme dosages. Rather ironic, don't you think? Sue Kelly was the nurse who came to the house to show both John and me how to set up the IV. If I hadn't experienced this at the Adams Center, it would have been very complicated. My treatments were to be twice a day for six to eight weeks which meant that I would have to awaken at 4:30 am with John for the "two man operation".

The next morning we sat at the kitchen table and when the IV was finished, John walked to the couch in the den with me, kissed me good-bye and left. What a long day it seemed to be and I was very tired and nervous. Home Care Services called to tell me about a change in the hook-up which someone would arrange on Thursday, and, also change the shunt and give a demo. Again, they recommended I find a LI doctor.

Following the same procedure the next day, which certainly beat being in a hospital for the IV, everything went well until I started with diarrhea that continued until the next day. When the nurse Kathy came, she put a new shunt in my arm, explaining it should last 14 days. Concerned about my diarrhea, she recommended the BRAT diet – (banana, rice, apple, toast) and Kaopectate, and, if not better, by the next day to call my physician or a Dr. Retolli in Huntington, a rheumatologist. I called Dr. Retolli and made an appointment for Friday at noon.

Feeling better on the BRAT diet but when the nurse came to change the IV site, she had a problem and after trying to do so too often, I started to black out. On the following day, March 1st, I completed my first week of the IV, but felt so drained.

During the afternoon of March 3rd, sudden pains in my mid-drift area and around to my back gripped me, lasting for about 15 minutes, leaving me scared because I knew it had to be a result of the IV.

Finally Friday arrived and I met with Dr. Retolli for over an hour telling him my story from the beginning. "You were taken; there is no such thing as CFS," he declared and told me the blood tests were bogus. Also questioning the Lyme tests, he nevertheless, told me to continue the IV, but only once a day for the 21 day accepted medical dosage. Pointing out the serious side effects and the results of over treatment for Lyme, I was shaking. His medical diagnosis was Fibromyalgia (a pain and fatigue syndrome) and as a result, he prescribed Flexeril once a day at bedtime.

Dr Retolli pushed the right buttons. I liked him, I believed him and I decided to go along with his treatment.

Immediately after the IV the very next day, I felt ill with chills and a 101 degree fever. A doctor on call at the Home Services told me to stop the IV after the next day (Sunday) and to call Dr. Retolli on Monday. After a bad night with pain again in my middle section, almost taking me to the emergency room, I was petrified to use the IV that day. My mind was a complicated whirl. Again, I thought if I leave Stein completely, could I count on Dr. Retolli?

On Monday Dr. Retolli's receptionist relayed my message to him and his answer was to stop the IV. I asked her to please have the doctor call me. Glad to stop the IV, yet the question, who is right, Stein or Retolli, hung in the balance?

After Barry and I talked on Thursday he called Jim Stein who in turn called me. At first, he wanted to give me the oral antibiotic, Biaxin, but backed off when I explained how Dr. Retolli felt about over treatment for Lyme. He asked me to take another urine test. I refused. In fact, at this point, I would not even take a pill without consulting Dr. Retolli. It will be through him that I will be able to reclaim my health, I convinced myself.

Less pain in both hips and feet was a tremendous relief although the constant tingling sensations and twitching in both legs continued. However, I could actually cook dinner and clean! Errands no longer overwhelmed me and I didn't collapse when I returned home. Judging my activities and giving myself enough time, I found that I could create enough balance so that my objectives would be met and my physical and emotional well being rewarded by a "job well done".

On the day before St. Patrick's Day I received a letter from the Lindenhurst School District inquiring if I planned to return in September. Our letters must have crossed; I had already sent them a letter saying I planned to return.

Sometime, in between the IV's and the Flexeril, I was beginning to regain my health! The first indication was not feeling so fatigued. A major improvement indeed for it was the heavy lethargy that kept me from functioning at work and even at home. Cautious at first, yet slowly and surely, much longer periods of stamina sustained me.

No longer on a strict diet but eating healthy foods and walking for exercise on a far limited schedule, I felt that a slower pace combined with an "everything in moderation" attitude was the road to take. Lounging in the sun, drinking herbal tea, reading and meditating became a normal pampered part of my life!

So on St. Patrick's Eve while the corned beef and cabbage were simmering, much to my delight, I sat in the kitchen, and added up all my medical bills for 1992. The total was a whopping $10,000 and that was with double coverage; John's and mine. Of course, some of the doctors I used wouldn't be covered under any plans!

On March 18th when Jim Stein called I reminded him that I still hadn't received my urine test results. "They're on the way," he said; reminded me of "the check is in the mail". I also told him that 50% of my fatigue was gone! He was thrilled and felt that we were on the right track. "Think we may have killed the critters," he laughed, but to "undo the damage" more anti-biotics through IV or orally may be needed. Another bacterium could be involved, he also felt, but could be treated the same way. The relief I felt knowing I was better lent credence to anything he said, and I hoped Dr. Retolli would be as cooperative.

The joy I felt on the first day of spring since I had made it through the winter was like no other spring I could remember. I could hardly wait for my appointment with Dr. Retolli the next day.

No more anti-biotics and take 1 1/2 Flexeril - 15 mg. were his orders. He also wrote a prescription for physical therapy. Return in 5 weeks. Again, he told me the urine test was bogus. Yet, I had to know and would take it to Plainview. It was time to say good-bye to Dr. Jim Stein.

It wasn't until the last week of April that Jim and I spoke. The Urine Test for Lyme was O+34. Suggesting I take more vitamins and oils, he asked when I was going to celebrate.

"I'm planning to throw myself a big party, will you come?" I asked him. Jim would try to and let me know. My excitement kept my happy thoughts spinning that night. It didn't matter that I could hardly sleep!

Chapter 22

TURNING POINT

Slowly, but surely, I was getting better. It no longer mattered who was right and who was wrong. Dr. Stein insisted I had Lyme disease, Dr. Retolli said it was, and is, Fibromyalgia.

I continued taking Flexirl at bedtime during the entire spring and summer and into the fall. Twice a week, for six weeks, deep tissue massage, and stretching and strengthening my muscles was my Physical Therapy regime and I continued to take vitamins and homeopathic medicine as well. Yes, there were ups and downs, but generally, I was well on my way to recovery.

It was still a mystery to me as to why the alternative doctor prescribed the most powerful medicine (strong antibiotics in IV form; twice the dosage a traditional doctor would prescribe). If the blood work for Lyme wasn't reliable, how could a doctor tell a patient she had Lyme?

On the other hand, in 1993 when I started researching Fibromyalgia, it was not well known or understood by most physicians. Very few people had ever heard of it. I read that it was a form of "arthritis of the muscles with no known cure, with its symptoms so varied, widespread and vague". Since there were no real observable and definitive tests, it was more

99

like a game of take away, ruling out other more frightening illnesses with X-rays, MRI'S, blood tests, etc.

So what! Who cares? I want to live again! It was time to celebrate!

Chapter 23
CELEBRATION

I kept telling myself that I would throw a party and invite all the people who came into my life during the time I was so very sick. They were the people who deserved to celebrate with me. It was a way in which to show them my gratitude for putting up with me.

One of my art teacher friends designed the lovely invitations with hand sketched seashells and beach grass. Here it is..................

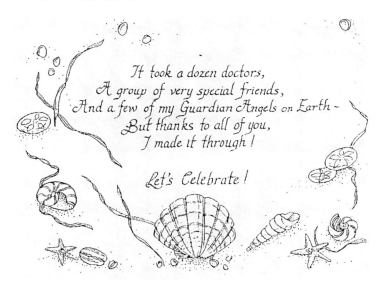

*It took a dozen doctors,
A group of very special friends,
And a few of my Guardian Angels on Earth –
But thanks to all of you,
I made it through!*

Let's Celebrate!

102 | *Gail Wench*

I planned to fill in the date as soon as I knew when Jim Stein would be flying to New York from Arizona. Couldn't have the celebration without him!

Finally, I mailed the invitations and was so amazed that most all of the forty people would attend, including Jim Stein, Dr. B., Dr. Barbara Sloan, Barry Clark, Clara, and several close friends.

And so on Saturday, July 31st at 5pm at our home, in our back yard, set with tables and chairs and beautiful pink tablecloths, napkins, and gorgeous flowers, John and I were ready to welcome our guests. The Beggar's Banquet, of course, arranged the wonderful hot and cold buffet.

For this "historic" occasion, I wanted to wear a dress that was perfect; not too dressy but not too casual. Happily, I found the perfect dress! It was coral in color with wide straps, designed like a sarong. I loved it and with multi-colored sandals, I felt like a movie star!

Both John and I loved introducing everyone. They might have been strangers to some, but to us, they were our guardian angels. Everyone was here for one purpose and that was the miracle that bonded us all. That beautiful evening under the twinkling star-studded sky ended all too soon.

Resting at the beach the next day, John and I said to one another, "Did last night really happen or was it just a dream?" We both agreed it was a 'Magical Night' and one we wouldn't forget for the rest of our lives!

Chapter 24

HALLEHUJAH

Yes, I was physically ready to go back to work in September 1993!

The other question; was I mentally ready, well, sort of.

Greeted warmly, especially by the principals, I was a bit reticent with some of the faculty and not as outgoing as I had been before my sick leave. My classes were filled with receptive students, for which I was very grateful, as well as the schedule I was given. My appreciation for all that I had previously taken for granted was truly a visible blessing.

Imagine finding my classroom looking exactly the same as when I had left it almost two school years ago! This time around, a high stool which I covered in a bright turquoise fabric helped me when standing became too difficult, and gave me enough height so that my eyes could see into every corner of the room.

Slowly but surely, I was back in the swing of things, like a bike rider who never forgets how to ride even after a mighty fall. Bea walked again with me as if we'd never stopped. How fortunate I was to have all the horror behind me.

Yet, Dr. Retolli still prescribed Flexeril and my telephone connection with Dr. Stein continued. Everyone once in awhile, I would wean myself off the Flexeril, only to discover

103

that I had to resume it, since episodes of muscle pain in my legs and hips had not stopped entirely.

Perhaps my appreciation and gratefulness for the stamina I was able to maintain helped me to tolerate the sporadic downside and led me to accept and enjoy the fact that I would probably never be the person I once was. Recalling the many people I had met, the unlikely experiences I encountered, and the new places I visited, broadened my small, tidy, regimented world. It was all that I had experienced these last two years that subtly changed and expanded my life.

Chapter 25

BLINK

Time sure flies when you're having fun! Where did all those years go? Here it was April 2006 and I just celebrated my 55th birthday, which for a teacher who has taught for thirty years, is a very significant age.

In spite of all the excesses and my illness, I accrued just over thirty years of teaching. It was the end of a six year contract and there was talk of RETIREMENT. Never would I have even said that word or much less thought about it. Yet, something told me, I'd better consider it when the offer was presented.

On one hand, I loved teaching and am proud to say that teaching was what I did best. My reputation as one of the finest teachers in the Middle School was an off- shoot, I liked to say, of blood, sweat and tears! Mentoring new teachers and conducting "Professional Circles" where groups of 2nd, 3rd and 4th year teachers met to discuss all sorts of phases of teaching, often in a "talk show", setting were activities that enriched our school district and gave me invaluable opportunities to stay at the top of my game.

How did it happen that not too many years ago I was one of the youngest teachers (31 years old) on the Middle School faculty; now I was one of the oldest? Yet, I bonded even more so with the younger generation, probably because of my counseling, and group seminars. But, truthfully, I was older and felt it. Perimenopausal, the doctor's called it, and, wouldn't you know, for me a side effect was insomnia.

Prior to this, after my usual busy days of teaching, meetings, working out and walking, cooking dinner and maintaining the usual household chores, I'd fall into bed at 9:00pm and sleep the sleep of a baby. Now, strings of sleepless nights led to anxious thoughts about my health.

And so, almost by rote, I dialed Dr. Retolli's number, the first time in several years, and made an appointment. Of course, he remembered me; with my story, how could he forget? After our catch-up chat, he prescribed Flexeril which would once again give the REM sleep I needed.

Inevitably, hot flashes interrupted my sleep and the insomnia persisted. Getting through the days became difficult. Was my body once again betraying me? Quality free time became non-existent; exhaustion reared its ugly head. The decision to make my decision to retire was what I knew I had to do. Fear that my life would "be over" if I left my profession added to my restless nights.

The dilemma would prey on my mind while I prayed for the right decision, and more than that, what could I do if I chose retirement?

For many days, the little voice in my head repeated, "Gail, there just may be something else out there for you; your life won't be over. At age fifty-five you certainly can still do something else!"

But what?

Chapter 26

NOT FOR SISSIES

I dove in, head first! My world was shocked, especially John! Here I was retired but my husband was not even able to consider retirement until he was sixty-two. With my life and pursuits almost surrounded by teaching, colleagues, students and friends could not understand my purpose of retiring.

After what I viewed as my endless summer, I put on "my big girl panties" and began to list the things I had promised myself that I would do in this - "my new life".

At first I increased my gym workouts, worked outdoors in my garden, and ate lunch on the weekdays at Glen's. Although these were singular activities, I did meet and chat with people, and before I knew it, friendships grew. Just a few here and a few there; some just a welcoming "hi" or "I saved you a seat Gail".

Like as a baby, I was exploring a world where I was seeking a new place to fit. Beyond my familiar province of teaching, I knew of very little. My sense of accomplishment on a daily basis in the classroom was a 'purpose-reward system' that I needed to continue.

Gratefully, I jumped at the chance to teach Adult Education two nights a week in Lindenhurst. The students were adults anxious to learn English. A teacher is a teacher, and, once again I took on a familiar role with a familiar purpose. Happily, I knew the staff; we bonded quickly. Working with adults who "sweated" long daytime hours in local factories or who cleaned offices and houses, my admiration for these folks was tremendous. Just as they did, I looked forward to each Tuesday and Thursday evening and regaled with them at the astonishing progress they made! Talk about accomplishments!

Now if only I could balance my health situation, as well as I had stabilized my need to function in a similar profession, I was determined to create the perfect mix. First of all, something had to be done to alleviate the nagging insomnia and hot flashes.

A new store called Healthy Alternatives offered acupuncture which I learned could help to lessen menopausal problems. Knowing myself, it wasn't very long before I decided to try acupuncture.

During my first visit I was enchanted with the beautiful décor, the delightful scented aromatherapy essences that seemed to float through the shop, and the friendly staff. Shari, my acupuncturist and I bonded immediately. Yet, eventually, the procedure didn't help and my erratic sleep patterns resulted in my going back to bed on the mornings I felt so tired.

Another appointment with Dr. Retolli; another prescription for Flexeril. Long overdue for a mammography and my yearly gynecological exam, my promises to take better care of myself, now that retirement gave me the time, were in vain. Was I just all talk and no action?

Chapter 27
DÉJÀ VU

Not that much had changed during my first year of retirement. Teaching ESL two nights a week, tutoring once a week, working out, and walking for exercise was the extent of the "new me".

Was I frittering away the year? Was it okay to enjoy my quiet times of reading and playing with my ten year old little girl, Missy, our five pound mini-Chihuahua, who in reality replaced the baby John and I never had and who was the light of our lives?

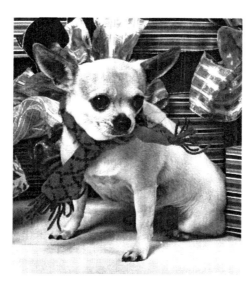

Was I in a rut? For the first time since I began my teaching career and with the exception of the almost two years I was so sick, enjoying my home on a daily basis was a definite new situation in my life. No longer did I rush to leave my home in the morning, rush home to have dinner and rush out again to meetings with my thoughts a whirlwind of students, lessons, exams, faculty meetings etc. So it was during this year while I felt so much better that my time spent at home became pretty darn valuable to me.

Would you believe that Missy and I watched "our favorite TV shows" together? It was on Oprah one day that I caught a loud and clear message. A Dr. Oz discussed facing one's fear by making the necessary doctor appointments to ensure good health. Recent symptoms of heart palpitations, that I thought were related to menopause, helped me to make the GYN appointment with Dr. Judd very quickly; in fact, immediately after the show!

My appointment was on Halloween; no costumes in this office! Dr. Judd, very nice and so kind, took my blood pressure again after reading the number his intern had recorded. It was incredibly high. He considered sending me to the hospital, but I interrupted and explained that I had "White Coat Syndrome" which spikes my blood pressure count whenever I am in a doctor's office. The good doctor took it again; it had lowered a bit. However, still concerned he asked me to see a doctor in Bay Shore, ASAP, and to also purchase a BP kit as soon as I left the office.

The Bay Shore doctor was not taking any new patients, his receptionist told me, and, no, she could not recommend any other doctor. Even at home my blood pressure was very high as I saw for myself.

Following Dr Judd's advice, when he gave me the name of a Dr. Richard Berber in Massapequa, I drove to the address given to me and pulled up in front of a little house, sitting in the middle of an over-grown front yard, with a sign that read Dr. Richard Berber, D.O. and almost kept right on driving. Was Dr. Judd crazy? I thought the doctor to whom I was to see was a cardiovascular man, not an osteopath!

Somehow I very reluctantly managed to go inside. The receptionist sat in an amazingly clean room and couldn't have been more welcoming. Dr. Berber listened patiently to my story and when I told him I had "White Coat Syndrome", he replied with a twinkle in his eyes, "Don't worry, my coat is tattle-tail gray!"

Right off the bat, I knew I was going to like this doctor. My blood pressure was high; tattle-tail gray was added to the list of syndromes. He set up an appointment for a corroded artery exam and advised me to wear a heart monitor but to go about my regular schedule. Feeling quite comfortable with this doctor, I just knew I'd be okay, yet, I would be in for a few surprises!

Chapter 28

WHAT'S UP DOC?

After I returned the heart monitor to Dr. Berber's office, I went to tutor Samantha, and returned home just before dinnertime. John had beaten me home and as I walked in, he casually mentioned that I had a voice mail from a doctor.

"What doctor, what did he say?" I said as I rushed to the phone. Dr. Berber's message said I needed to call him immediately; it was urgent. Now what? What could be wrong?

The results from my heart monitor test, Dr. Berber said, necessitate that I come to see him the next morning. Apparently, my blood pressure was extremely high in the early morning hours, a time when a heart attack or stroke is most likely.

I was so unnerved by that conversation that I could almost hear my heart beating like a drum. John helped me, or rather John cooked dinner, while I babbled on about my fears. Of course, you must have guessed by now that I didn't sleep a wink that night!

Once again John took a day off from work to drive me to the doctor's office. I truly was terrified. After checking my blood pressure again, making a few calls and filling out forms, Dr. Berber directed me to a cardiologist in Amityville.

Both doctors agreed on further testing and medication. My life style, they felt, was not indicative of someone who had high blood pressure. Yet, it was the #1 killer of middle aged women and very often undiagnosed. Maybe, I was saved in the nick of time!

After a few more visits I began to reflect upon the irony of it all. Years ago when I had Lyme/Fibromyalgia I could not find a doctor to treat me. Now, here I was in 2007, feeling pretty good, yet focused upon, because of high blood pressure; the silent killer. Thinking about those many years of being a guinea pig, it was very interesting to note all the changes in the medical field during these past fifteen years.

Test results could now measure my illness. No longer was I a part of the unknown; I had a legitimate illness. Almost like being on a pedestal, I noticed how the doctors and their staff treated me very respectfully. No one rushed me out the door. Instead, my health and I both were of seemingly genuine interest; a far cry from years ago.

There were no side effects to my blood pressure medication! What a joy and relief it was to pursue my daily activities and actually plan ahead safely. Ever so thankful, my plans for Thanksgiving and Christmas rolled merrily along!

Chapter 29

IT'S NOT OVER

In January of 2008 I had my six months check up appointment with Dr. Retolli and decided to bring my test results along with my latest health issues to keep him aware of my most recent developments. Although he was a specialist in rheumatology, I trusted his overall knowledge and expert advice. At the very least, he was a good listener!

After reviewing my blood test results and the other reports, he informed me that he was on the Board of Directors at Huntington Hospital and continued to say that he would be outraged if any of his staff came to him with my symptoms and no more tests.

Needless to say, I was taken back not only by his words but also by the tone of his voice. Finally, I stuttered, "Wh-wh-what do-do you mmm-mean?"

"Gail," replied Dr. Retolli,"you definitely need more blood work and you must go for a renal artery sonogram." Pausing a few moments, he continued. "Gail, what I have just told you is standard procedure. How in the world could an osteopath and a cardiologist miss that?"

Letting that, too, sink in before he went on, "Gail, you are in too good a shape with your diet and your exercise program to be exhibiting such high blood pressure counts. Therefore,

115

in my opinion," he said very slowly, "there has to be another cause."

"Uh- oh," I was starting to sweat, thinking, what does he know that the others don't know? How can this be? Now what?

The upshot included more blood work, more blood tests, more calls to Dr. Retolli's busy office and finally after a few months with no clear cut reasons to be found, he recommended that I see one of the doctors he knew, a Dr. Olnut, a hypertension expert at Huntington Hospital.

I felt as terrible as someone who had won the lottery, and now it was being taken away, forcing the person to return to a life of misery. The idea and the thought of running back and forth again from doctor to doctor, diagnosis upon diagnosis to be reversed, changed, questioned, and God knows what else, just might put me right back into the middle of a world of craziness and crazies. Hadn't I been in the medical rabbit hole long enough?

Like a puppet, I made the call to his colleague. At first I was told there would be several weeks wait and so I hung up the phone. Minutes later I got a call; I could be seen the next evening. (Dr. Retolli had called in my behalf).

The symptoms of terrifying fear began again. "Face Your Fears Gail", I repeated over and over to myself.

I dreaded telling my Adult Ed Program supervisor that I would not be coming in that night. First of all, to let my students down made me very sad and to break my perfect attendance record punctured my ego.

With my dear John at the wheel, we found the address of the new doctor easily. What a coincidence to be right next to the Huntington Mall. "Let's shop afterwards," I half-heartedly teased John.

This new office of kidney specialists included Dr. Olnut as one of the three team doctors. Maybe I have a rare kidney disease, I thought. After all, my father died from kidney problems when he was in his fifties.

My blood pressure, true to its state of alarm, was "off the charts". Why hadn't my new medication netted results? Dr. Olnut's Turkish accent was as charming as his smile, but, of course, he didn't go for "The White Coat Syndrome". Instead, he changed and increased my medication, and made arrangements for more blood work and tests.

As usual I went along for the ride. At one point Dr. Olnut and Dr. Retolli thought my high blood pressure was caused by the renal artery but further tests proved otherwise. In fact, no single cause was found.

Continuing to see Dr. Olnut every few weeks, then once a month, then every three months until only every six months, I came to realize that he, of all the others, was the perfect doctor! There was so much about him and his surroundings that made me feel comfortable. Not having to wait to see him was a godsend. I felt that the friendly staff and bright, clean office reflected his consideration of his patients.

There wasn't a single visit when I felt rushed or that I couldn't discuss something on my mind. In fact, Dr. Olnut listened patiently to everything I told him, whether it was about health issues or something else going on in my life. He made me feel that what I had to say was interesting and important.

After all these years of doctors, other than Dr. Retolli who saved my life, (got to love him) and Drs. Judd and Berber, it was Dr. Olnut who ended my search for the perfect doctor.

And as far as my darn old high blood pressure, maybe I'd look into using alternative medicine again.

Chapter 30

OD'ED ON YOGA

Several of my gym friends and I had been practicing Yoga every Saturday and Sunday morning at our local gym. Starting as beginners but after four years becoming serious students, we were considered to have reached the intermediate level of an athletic-style Yoga. Unlike meditation and breathing regimes, our level, especially for me was quite a challenge due to my tight muscles and stiff lower back and hips. Yet I knew it was good for me, as I felt physically and emotionally better after each workout.

Gladys, one of my favorite instructors, encouraged me to join LIYA (Long Island Yoga Association) which gave monthly workshops and weekend retreats. Taking her advice, for I certainly had the time now during retirement, I did. There was no doubt about it; I was extremely involved in Yoga!

As an avid reader, who enjoyed fiction and non-fiction equally, I seemed to be gravitating now toward spiritual and self-discovery themed books, some of which had been Oprah recommendations; others from Healthy Alternatives. At the time of my first Yoga retreat, *The Power of Now,* by Eckart Tolles, was my book of choice.

Even though I did have reservations about leaving John and Missy for the weekend retreat, my reading had given me a sense of adventure, new experiences and the idea of acting in the now, and so Gladys and another Yoga enthusiast, Lisa, a great lady, joined me for the weekend at Brentwood's St. Joseph Renewal Center.

As a former Catholic girls' boarding school, and now a home for some of the older nuns, as well as a private day care center, and nursing facility, it was still maintained by the Catholic Church. When Lisa and I arrived late that Friday afternoon, we marveled at the beautiful grounds that seemed to go on forever. Actually, the center was on at least 100 acres of land. As we drove along the long, winding gravel road to what I can only describe as the hotel from Stephen King's, *The Shining*, I was spooked! Only minutes away from home, yet we had entered another time zone.

Massive on the outside as well as the inside, with endlessly long hallways, high ceilings, towering staircases, and dark curling shadows, I shivered and whispered to Lisa, "My God, where are we?" Crammed into a tiny elevator (the only small thing we had yet seen), we finally arrived at the fourth floor and found our rooms. In the space of a closet, there was a single bed, a small desk and a lamp; nothing else. A community bathroom with showers was down the hall; an immaculately clean area but, oh, so very hot. Even my opened one window had no effect. It remained hot; only the showers were cold.

After we had checked out the large meeting room, where we would be practicing several types of Yoga with various instructors, we found the basement cafeteria. Unfortunately, I soon learned that the quality of the food was inedible. I had come here for the Yoga experience, I kept reminding myself, not a four star hotel.

The instructors and the participants fascinated me as did the new styles of Yoga. The closest I got to read my book was glancing at it on my lap. Interestingly, Gladys encouraged me to pay attention to any feelings I might be experiencing; physically or emotionally.

"What do you mean?" I couldn't imagine what she was talking about. She didn't reply. We continued to practice meditation, chanting and breathing and tried new techniques. As much as I enjoyed my three days, I missed my little Missy and John, and was very excited to leave for home on Sunday afternoon.

Chapter 31

LIVING IN THE NOW

Missy and John were waiting outside for my arrival. While John looked as happy to see me as I did seeing him, I scooped up my little girl and wouldn't let go. Only two and a half days away from home and I ran inside yelling, "There's no place like home!"

As if I'd been away for a year, staying in a drab place, I seemed to be looking at our house for the first time. Walking all around, I began focusing on my favorite things, and catching the sunlight sparkling through the windows, highlighting the furniture and soft colors of the décor, was pure enchantment. Hungry, or rather starving and tired, we ordered in; food never tasted as good as it did this night!

My five senses were alive and incredulously heightened. Could this be an affect of the retreat? Whatever it was, a new target had surfaced.

Choosing not to watch TV or talk on the phone, instead I took a lovely, warm bath, snuggled into bed with Missy and John (no book) and slept like a rock.

Waking up to a bright, glorious sunlit bedroom, I got up slowly, didn't rush off to the gym or even take a walk. After John left for work, Missy and I sat outside at her favorite spot. I picked up *The Power of Now* but quickly put it down. I needed

123

to take in the new spring air, the extra deep green of the grass, our brightly colored flowers, the chirping of the birds and even in the distance the sounds of a lawnmower humming. I even listened to my neighbors talking and laughing. Was this really Gail or someone else so attuned to all that surrounded her?

THEN, I began to read. After the introduction I put the book down for a moment....... I was literally experiencing the very POWER of now of which the author was writing - living in the moment - just BEING! It was astounding to me; I was blown away. All because of the Yoga Retreat? Was this what Gladys was trying to tell me?

For the next five days, my living in the present miraculously held. In fact, my positive feelings inspired me to do things previously just thought about for so long. First, I returned to Healthy Alternatives, telling the group of my experience at the retreat and the way in which Tolles' book had affected me.

Donna, the owner, was so intrigued that she said to me, "Gail, I've been looking for someone to host a book club," to which I replied eagerly," I've been looking for someone to hire me since I retired. I would love to run a book club, a self-discovery book club!"

This was just what I needed; I was flying high! When I went back to the gym later that day I even spoke to the owner about a yoga workshop similar to the retreat. He was delighted. Wow! To think I had landed two jobs in one day was absolutely amazing!

It didn't take me long to gather a group of thirty five women who agreed to meet at my favorite restaurant, Lucy's Café, on a very hot June evening, for our very first book session.

Living in the Now | 125

Talking about my experiences because of *The Power of Now* turned out to be the recipe for a successful first meeting.

Preparing as carefully and concentrating on a well-planned and organized agenda, the yoga workshop also was a success. To my astonishment, I had arranged and executed two groups that I believed would help others, while blessing me with healthy goals.

Chapter 32

FINDING BALANCE

Of course, I would tell everyone I ran into about my yoga workshop and new book club; you couldn't shut me up!

That fall, Lisa and I returned to St. Joseph's Renewal Center for a weekend of Buddhist study bringing along two friends, Mary and Alinson. (I later discovered that *The Power of Now* and Buddhism had many similarities.) The first night we were to observe something called NOBLE SILENCE. "What's that?" we all asked at once.

There would be no speaking for twelve hour stretches. "No way will I do this," one of the girls remarked. But I did it! Not sure how, but since I had spent many long periods of time at home alone, often meditating, reflecting and reading, it wasn't as difficult as I thought it would be, especially since my book club selections helped to put me on my own self-discovery journey. Quiet, thoughtful and peaceful times were now part of my daily routine instead of a fast-paced, spur of the moment existence.

However, my blood pressure was still high, even though my blood work results, Dr. Olnut informed me, were good. The same old "sky high" numbers appeared whenever Dr. O took my pressure. Once he sent another doctor in to take it; it decreased only slightly.

127

Resting, breathing deeply, even music did nothing to lower my pressure. Oh well, complaining was no longer my style. Too many other people had serious illnesses that they accepted with such grace, so who was I to fuss?

Often thinking of my favorite President Teddy Roosevelt's quote,

"Do what you can, with what you have, where you are," so simple and yet profound, tweaked my evaluation of my endeavors. Am I doing everything I can, in every situation in which I am placed? And; if so, good. Practice just BEING each day, I would remind myself. Each encounter, even with strangers, I learned matters, for it is in all kinds of experiences that one receives the chance to share.

Chapter 33

IS LIFE BEAUTIFUL?

On my way to Lucy's Café for a coffee and yogurt each morning, I would walk along an alley-way where a window sign read *Life Is Beautiful Chiropractic Office*. Signs like that sure do have a positive reaction; a sort of 'come hither' nuance. The owner would often be at Lucy's getting his coffee, too, and I had been introduced to him as Dr. John Balsamo who happened to be a friend of my friend, Jackie.

Since my long relationship with chiropractors ended about fifteen years ago, I thought it time to visit Life Is Beautiful. Unlike any office I had ever been in, Dr. Balsamo's included a big, black Labrador called Sal, who greeted patients at the door. On one wall was a hand-painted beach mural which also referenced many of the doctor's many interests.

An aura of friendliness and relaxation permeated this office. Certainly I was headed in the right direction! In each room there were two tables and if two patients were not there, Sal would wander in and lie down next to the empty table or even stroll in, wag his tail and stop for a petting. "Bizzare," you exclaim, "for a doctor's office!

Get past all that; grow up!

I felt that this office just might have offered the most relaxing atmosphere and given the best care I had received in a very long time. It didn't take much to persuade John and Missy to come with me! The gathering of family, friends and clients that continually walked into Dr. John's office became a part of my life, of our life.

Somehow, I knew it was meant to be.

When I mentioned my book to Dr J. and told him that I had included him and his wonderful office in Chapter 33, he looked surprised and then explained, "Chapter 33 Gail? Did you know that there are 33 principals of Chiropractic treatment? And, did you know that Christ died at the age of 33?"

I just smiled.

There is a new sign in the office now (among other words of wisdom) that reads:

PLEASE DO NOT ASK US MEDICAL QUESTIONS

Medical doctors are wrong 4 out of 10 times.* We are not medical doctors and will be wrong 10 out of 10 times and will surely kill you. We will not be responsible for your death.

PLEASE DO ASK US CHIROPRACTIC QUESTIONS

Because we are experts on Chiropractic and would love to answer Chiropractic questions, thereby improving (and maybe even saving) your life.

*JAMA, December 21, 1994, Vol. 272, No. 23, "error in Medicine"

Is chiropractic medicine working for us? Will it help lower my blood pressure? Will it increase our quality of life as well as longevity? We're working on it!

Chapter 34

A SERENDIPITOUS JOURNEY

For years just to say the word Fibromyalgia was too painful. Those agonizing years were behind me. The journals I painstakingly kept were put away and gathering dust. The book I had started so long ago remained untouched. How grateful I was to leave the past where it belonged and to focus on the NOW which had finally captured me.

Strangely enough, however, more and more signs and reasons cropped up, urging me to complete my book. Even though few people had heard of "my disease" which had only been diagnosed in 1990 and took until 2009 to become an often spoken word, because of the glut of commercials, the concern and interest was apparent.

Perhaps my experiences would be of help to others. After all, I laughed to myself; I was a wealth of information! And since I had definitely crossed the line between living my affliction and moving forward, I felt I had much to offer. Surely, there were times when a change of plans was necessary because I didn't feel as well as I would have liked, (oh well, that lousy old "f-word" again) but it was nothing like being lost in the maze of searching before I received a diagnosis.

It is said that Fibromyalgia, a common, complex chronic pain disorder affecting people physically, emotionally and socially is unlike a disease with a specific cause and recognizable symptoms.

In fact, it is still an enigma today, challenging traditional and alternative medicine, and taking several years, in some cases, to even diagnose. Because there is no current cure, a life-long life style of adaptation is one of the keys to progress. For me, not giving up during the most difficult episodes of my illness, would remind me of why I had held on for so long.

Learning to manage my situation and accepting the fact that I would never be "cured" I arrived at a point where I was able to speak more openly about this disease. If there was only one person I might help, I would feel tremendously rewarded. With the power of NOW and the knowledge, lessons, pain and experiences from yesterday, my personal resources and experiences were my gifts to share. So what if I wasn't the young, vibrant woman I was once. Through it all I found something worth far more than I was seeking.

That word; that word *serendipity*, a word I had to check for its exact meaning: stumbling, tripping toward the unexpected describes not only my arduous journey, but more importantly my discovery of many silver-lined clouds. I am also reminded of Mac and Simon looking from the overlook at the Grand Canyon, overwhelmed by its beauty, size and timelessness, and reflecting on our short earthly existence. Looking at the big picture and not sweating the small stuff has given me a life that makes all my experiences count.

My life is layered like a rock composed of many components, each of necessity to my strength. Each person, every encounter and experience is necessary and essential to my physical, emotional, and social balance. However the struggles of my determined quest, the serendipitous benefits are my salvation.

EPILOGUE

Something was in the air during the late spring of 2009, something unexplainable. I could feel it. As if I were on a fringed precipice, I knew that unforeseen events were about to occur. Our plans to do a major renovation on our home were in the works. Endless conversations, choosing a contractor, picking out all sorts of upgrades, deciding on colors, fabrics, paneling, paint, and carpeting frustrated, worried, baffled and eventually delighted us. Great expectations accompanied our decisions and we were on top of the world!

So thorough was our commitment to the renovation, we never planned for ourselves. How in the world could we live here during the utter turmoil? No sooner had our thoughts been expressed, when out of the blue, came a startling invitation from a new acquaintance, offering her beach house in Montauk for the month of May!

John and I knew no one in Montauk. The thoughts of being able to stay where we always felt was the most beautiful paradise were almost unimaginable. Missy in Montauk? To walk the sandy beaches, whenever we wanted, just a few hundred feet from the house? Why, what a totally miraculous gift had been given to us!

Each night before falling asleep, the thoughts of our soon to be vacation raced through my mind; my lips in a perpetual smile. With a time to relax and a special oasis to return to my book, my dreams were a whirl of scrambled excitement.

We were like kids playing in a doll's house from the moment we arrived at the beach house. Everything was so appropriate and evidently chosen with a Montauk theme. We oohed and aahed as we scurried from the living room and kitchen to the bedrooms and bathrooms finding all sorts of clever, quaint, colorful things that would surround us during our enchanting stay. Local newspapers, magazines, restaurant menus and all sorts of Montauk literature were there to our delight. John mentioned he saw an ad for a local editor, "someone you should meet honey," I thought I heard him say, as we were shuffling through the goodies.

Finding our way around the village and using the gazebo in the middle of the Village Green as our landmark, we discovered that so many roads that were filled with shops led right to the ocean. When John wanted to go to the tackle shop to get some surfcasting information, Missy and I tagged along and to our delight found a few plastic chairs outside the shop. Sitting in the warmth of the sun under the cloudless big blue sky, Missy and I almost fell asleep. It was so calm, so peaceful with just the slow swishing sounds of the waves. Imagine having a shop about 150' from the beach!

Shortly, as John walked out of Paulie's Tackle Shop followed by Paul, the owner and a small Asian man, a woman passed by and petted Missy. Everyone either sat on the stoop or a chair. It was as if the earth stood still; no one was in a hurry. Small chatter circled around Missy and then everyone was listening to me ramble on how we came to be in Montauk. Somehow introductions were made and, John, out of the blue said, "Aren't you the Real Estate agent who is also an editor?" to the woman called Eugenia. "I saw your ad and photo in the Montauk Pioneer and I told Gail she should meet you; Gail is writing a book you know."

BINGO!

The moment the connection was made, the small group listened intently to 'my story'. When I mentioned my book club and how anxious I was to someday send my book (if I ever completed it) to Oprah, the weather-beaten Asian man, and legendary Montauk surfcaster, Jack Yee, said his daughter was a producer on the Oprah Show. How incredulous was this scenario! Here I was in the midst of a group of strangers who not only shared their space with friendship but were also interested in my book. Instinctively, I knew that Eugenia would become my editor and friend. She would be the one to inspire me to finish what I had begun so long ago.

Just as Shelley told me so many years ago, we all have the power to hear what our heart is telling us. Sitting in Montauk like Shelley, listening to the rustling sounds of the waves, something told me I would complete what I had begun just as I had concentrated on changing my life.

As for my fourteen doors and my mattress, would I change them again? What do you think?

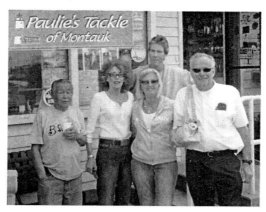